LIFEGIFTS

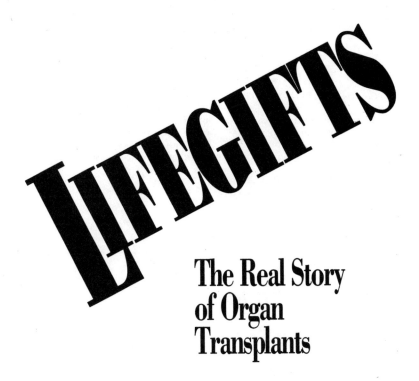

LIFEGIFTS

The Real Story of Organ Transplants

CALVIN STILLER M.D.

WITH

BRIAN C. STILLER

Stoddart

First published in 1990 by
Stoddart Publishing Co. Limited
34 Lesmill Road
Toronto, Canada
M3B 2T6

CANADIAN CATALOGUING IN PUBLICATION DATA

Stiller, C.R. (Calvin R.)
    Lifegifts

ISBN 0-7737-2301-3

1. Transplantation of organs, tissues, etc.
I. Title.

RD120.7.S84 1990   617'.95   C89-090624-6

Text illustrations: Louise Gadbois
Editing: Sara Swartz, Jane McNulty
Typesetting: Tony Gordon Ltd.

The author gratefully acknowledges permission to reprint:

The Human Tissue Gift Act, 1986; Ontario Ministry of the Solicitor
General. © Reprinted with permission from the Queen's Printer for
Ontario.

The Council of the Transplantation Society's guidelines for cadaver
organ distribution and living unrelated kidney donation. Reprinted
with permission of the Council of the Transplantation Society, London, England.

Printed and bound in the United States of America

To those donor families whose love for life and
thoughtfulness of others resulted in a lifegift

and to those whose life and health depend exactly
on that — our patients

C O N T E N T S

ACKNOWLEDGMENTS

This book could not have been written without the tireless and insightful editing (and harassment) of my brother Brian and the encouragement of my dear friend Bill Brady and his help in writing two of the chapters. Brian's extraordinary capacity to simplify the language and, along with editors Sarah Swartz and Donald G. Bastian, keep the book appropriate to the readership amazed me. If this book is received and the story understood by the public it is only because they overcame my natural tendencies to wander down sideroads and speak in medical jargon. The research and critical detailing of the text by Cate Abbott was so kindly but firmly contributed.

Through it all my personal colleagues showed toleration and gave me strong encouragement. The administration of the University Hospital, University of Western Ontario and Robarts Research Institute were kind and supportive.

It is not without some careful thought that I have included stories of my colleagues and patients to illustrate the points being made. This is not a traditional way for active physicians to write, but my patients have individually consented to this because of the hoped-for result: that the public will better understand the current potential of transplantation while grasping the correctable tragedy of wasted donor organs.

Time to write this book has largely been taken from my wife Angie, our family Cindy, Robert, Denice, Troy, Debi and Tim, and my extraordinary mother. I thank them for their indulgence — but also for the excitement they have shown for the project.

If only one donor is motivated, only one patient waiting for an organ encouraged, only one hospital board energized to enact an organ donor policy, the contributions of all the above will have been truly acknowledged!

INTRODUCTION

Traditionally, medicine has been limited to repairing the diseased body either by enhancing the normal healing process with medicines or by correcting defects with surgery. Prior to transplants, when someone was suffering from a fatal heart disease, the medical response all too often was, "Sorry, the heart is too badly damaged. There is nothing more we can do."

Transplants have allowed a second chapter to be written in the lives of critically ill patients. Instead of progressive disability or untimely death, the patient can now receive a new lease on life with a used but healthy organ to replace the diseased one.

My desire to help pioneer organ transplants had its beginnings in 1950. My father, a church minister, was ill with what was diagnosed as terminal kidney disease. A Mennonite physician, Dr. Abe Dyck, visited our prairie home often and became a friend of the family. I was so impressed with this man, I decided at the age of ten to become a doctor.

As a young medical student at the University of Saskatchewan in the early 1960s, I became interested in organ transplants. There was no place in the world where one could go for clinical training in this area, so we learned where we were, by doing.

Even as a student I believed that organ transplantation would, with the advent of new immunosuppressive agents, move from research to treatment for people with diseased hearts, livers, lungs and kidneys. Since kidney transplants were the only ones being done at that time, the best route, I decided, was to become a nephrologist — a kidney specialist.

The focus in those days was not so much on transplants as on tissue typing. I worked for Dr. Charles Baugh as a research technician at the University of Saskatchewan. He had returned from Johns Hopkins Hospital in Baltimore where they were attempting to tissue type a human in order to understand why patients who received a blood transfusion of the proper blood group would still react and become ill.

During the summer of 1962 I worked in the research building in which a Japanese plastic surgeon was achieving reasonable success with liver transplants in calves. This gave me the opportunity to observe an actual organ transplant.

In 1963, a two-year-old baby was brought in with biliary atresia, a condition from birth in which the bile ducts are not formed. Could a transplant save her? At that time there had never been a successful liver transplant. When a donor became available, an attempt was made. The outcome, however, was inevitable. The baby died. I was struck with the anguish of it all. Doctors had attempted to save a life without sufficient knowledge or research to ensure a reasonable chance of success.

In 1965, I moved to London, Ontario to complete my medical internship. During this time, a kidney transplant was carried out between two brothers, an event that attracted a great deal of publicity. As in the case of the liver transplant, this operation also failed, again because of insufficient research on which to base a successful outcome.

While still in training, I became involved with transplants at Victoria Hospital in London. I watched the usual course of events. A patient with diseased kidneys would live a miserable existence, surviving on the early and rather crude artificial kidney machine. A transplant would be carried out, usually without any major surgical problems. The kidney would function in the patient for a few days and the patient would get better. Then the inevitable fever would take over, followed by a look of panic on the face of the patient when he realized that something was wrong. Lethal drugs, necessary to suppress the rejection, would be given, against the odds that they would kill the patient. Sadly, most patients did die, either because the kidney was rejected or their bodies were overwhelmed by infection as a result of the drugs.

While these experiences were difficult, they were not totally discouraging. I became committed to combatting the obstacles to successful transplants. I was astounded by the trust that patients place in their physician, in their desperate bid for a cure and the extension of life.

In the fall of 1972, Dr. Wilder Penfield — professor of neurosurgery, director of the Montreal Neurological Institute and one of the greatest brain scientists in the world — opened the University Hospital in London, Ontario. In his address he challenged the hospital staff, in the words of Tennyson, "to strive, to seek, to find."

Dr. Ramsay Gunton, in charge of hiring staff, made a bold move. Instead of choosing a seasoned, experienced specialist to head up an organ transplant unit, he selected me, an unproven kid from Saskatchewan. The same fall that the University Hospital was established, we admitted our first patients.

Although I was a nephrologist by training, transplants were my real interest. I believed the answer to kidney failure would not be provided by an artificial kidney. I renewed my commitment to be able to offer patients transplants before they became sick and needed dialysis, or died.

Our hospital started out with a small, dedicated team who had on their side a hospital administration that believed, right from the beginning, that the success of the organ transplant program required research and experimentation, which eventually enabled us to move quickly from the laboratory to the bedside.

When we began, we knew the common enemy was tissue rejection. Our primary goal was to bridge the laboratory to the clinic, and the specialists of organ-related medicine to organ-related surgery. As a team leader, I learned that my role as chief of the unit — along with those doing transplant research, those who managed the organ donation and retrieval section, the specialists treating rejection, and ultimately, the surgical team — was to maintain the spirit and commitment of the team to retrieve every possible source of life from a donor body and to ensure that someone in need received the organ and experienced new life.

Chiefs of transplant units have traditionally been surgeons. The great pioneers of clinical transplantation have also been surgeons — David Hume, J. P. Murray, Tom Starzl, Sir Roy Calne, Norman Shumway and Christiaan Barnard. In my case, as an internist, I saw an opportunity to experience both the surgical and medical sides working hand in glove, for I knew that with transplants in particular, good surgery without good medicine would be just as fatal as good medicine without good surgery.

The board of directors and the medical advisory and management committees of the hospital have given their full support to transplantation. As a result, today we have the medical, technical, nursing and related expertise for a full-fledged, multi-organ transplant program — the first of its kind in Canada and one of a handful in the world.

Transplant surgery is almost always an emergency. Staff members are required to work under stressful conditions. Disruption of schedules is the rule. There is a personal price to pay: health care professionals ride emotional roller coasters not only with their patients before and after the transplant, but also with the donor families as they decide whether or not to donate the organs of their loved one.

Even so, organ transplants have become so common that society accepts them as a normal medical procedure. But there is so much we have yet to learn. In my journeys down the hospital halls, I have experienced extraordinary stories of life and death and have heard many questions that call for answers. I want to communicate this modern miracle of people reborn: the real story of organ transplants.

Good Luck, Bad Luck

ROBERT SEEMED THE MODEL of a good-looking, muscular 14-year-old — with one important exception. He lay propped up by pillows in a hospital bed. And over the quiet hiss of nasal oxygen, you could hear his desperate gasps for breath, the long inhalation characteristic of patients dying from heart failure, a symptom we call air hunger. Robert's skin was cold and moist. The bluish color of his hands indicated why it was difficult to arouse him: there was not enough blood going to his extremities or to his brain.

I didn't have to tell the parents that we had little time left. They knew. Just four days before, Robert (not real name) had been transferred to the University Hospital in London, Ontario from a hospital in Toronto. There, the medical team had done all they could in three previous heart operations. Robert had a congenital heart disease for which there was no surgical cure. The Toronto medical team had agreed that the only step that might save Robert's life would be a heart transplant. And since in 1984 they were not yet performing heart transplants at this hospital in Toronto, they were advised to seek assessment from our transplant center in London.

We examined Robert to see if he was eligible for a transplant. There was no question in the minds of the medical team that he was one of the sickest patients the London transplant team had ever assessed. He had been in heart failure for so long and his other organs had been so starved of blood that now the liver, kidneys and bowels were not functioning properly. We knew, however, that once the problem of inadequate blood supply had been solved, there would be a complete restoration of function in the other organs. A new heart could pump new life into Robert's entire body.

I looked at Robert and wondered if we hadn't been just a bit too quick to say yes. The boy was more ill than we had imagined. But there was no time to change our minds. The odds of Robert's survival no longer mattered because his probability of dying was 100 percent. A heart simply had to be found.

The size of the donor heart was very important. Since Robert was not a big boy, too large a heart would not fit his chest cavity and the size of the vessels would not match. This would cause turbulence in the circulatory system. We had to find a donor heart from a small woman or a child.

Our donor coordinator telephoned 24-ALERT, the donor-recipient matching system developed through NATCO (North American Transplant Coordinators Organization). (In 1986, UNOS — the United Network for Organ Sharing — was formed to be the comprehensive information center for those working in the transplant field. It's here that we both register our needs for organs and find out what is available and who else is waiting for a transplant.) The coordinator listened carefully to see whether there were any comparably urgent calls for a donor from any other center in North America. There were none. At least we would not be competing with another patient who was desperate for a donor heart. If another person had been listed in serious condition this would have complicated the problem of finding a suitable donor heart for Robert.

We dictated Robert's name into the computer system and assigned him an urgency rating of 9. At the time, that number signified that this patient would be dead in 24 hours if a donor were not found. (Since then a different rating system was instituted in North America.) We hoped there would be at least one potential donor, but there was none.

I turned to Michael Bloch, our senior transplant donor coordinator. He is the person who stays in touch with key medical staff and monitors the condition of the patient, which organs are available, where the organs are, and how they can be transported in time for a transplant. A transplant center simply cannot function without a transplant coordinator. There are too many procedures and people to organize in a critically short amount of time.

"Mike, get on the phone and call Pittsburgh, Minneapolis, Toronto and Atlanta. We're running out of time!"

Michael's calls started with the informal exchanges of friends from afar who never see each other but who talk every week, sharing an intense struggle against death. Each call ended with a thumbs up "We'll give you first chance at anything that comes up, Mike. Good luck."

Getting the right organ at the right time is still based solely on luck — good or bad luck. Had Robert come to our hospital the previous Saturday, he would have been in luck. At that time we had had a donor whose heart would have suited him perfectly. Today bad luck prevailed because there weren't any donors available anywhere on the eastern seaboard, as far west as Kansas City or as far south as Miami.

On the other hand, Robert's chance to live depended on someone else's bad luck. Somewhere, a small woman or a child about to die was Robert's only hope. How sadly ironic that someone's good luck was completely dependent on someone else's bad luck.

The first day passed into the second. Robert was now in kidney failure. His skin became jaundiced, telling us his liver was beginning to fail. The medical team conferred with Robert's mom and dad in the waiting room.

The darkening sky told me it was late in the afternoon. The hospital corridors were quiet. This was ski season and the ski buffs were taking advantage of the weather that weekend. But to

Robert's parents, one day of waiting was just like another. Their faces were stoic but their eyes betrayed terrible anxiety. They focused on the cardiologist's face. "I wish I could tell you that he's stable, but he's not," the cardiologist said. "I don't think he can last much longer."

The parents shifted their gaze to me. The father spoke. "Dr. Stiller, why can't you find a donor?" My professional exterior faltered. I could find some suitable medical explanation for almost any question, but in response to this one I had little to say.

I took the mother's hand and said quietly, "Mr. and Mrs. Peters, there just isn't a donor anywhere in central or eastern North America. I can assure you that if there was one, we would hear about it."

This was only a half-truth. Technically I was right: no donor had been located. I knew Michael Bloch had called every hospital and ICU (intensive care unit) he could find. But there *were* potential donors out there. Somewhere, amidst a population of more than 275 million, a child or small woman had died as a result of brain injury or brain hemorrhage. But either no one had asked for a donor heart, or someone had refused. We just didn't know how to locate this potential donor.

I knew there was one other way to find a donor, but it carried a high price. "Mrs. Peters," I said, "there is one further thing we can do, but I need your consent. We believe that somewhere out there is a potential donor. The only way we can stir people up to think about this is to launch a public appeal. You need to understand that this carries a personal price. If you go public and get an organ for Robert, the press will want to own you. They will demand details and invade your privacy for a long time. Yet they do a great job of blanketing the country. We know of no better way to reach people."

Mr. and Mrs. Peters are very private people. They had handled the serious illness of their son in private and they had decided to accept his impending death in private. Now their clear preference was to find a private solution.

Dr. Neil McKenzie, the cardiac surgeon, interpreted the distress on their faces. In his soft Scottish brogue, he said, "I think we could wait until tomorrow to decide this." We then agreed that if by five o'clock the next afternoon a donor had not been found, we would launch a public appeal.

We left the waiting room, and as we rounded the corner, Neil growled, "Dammit, I wish they had come a week earlier."

"Bad luck," commented Dr. Bill Kostuk, chief of cardiology.

There it was again! What should luck have to do with a matter of life and death? I wondered.

I left the hospital, unconsciously putting my hand to my belt and the ever-present pocket pager. With a quick press of my thumb, I tested it. The sharp beep told me the battery was good.

That night I had dinner with friends in a noisy restaurant. I tried unsuccessfully to take my mind off Robert. Twice I telephoned Michael. The weariness in his voice told me all: he had heard nothing. I advised him to get some sleep, because if we did find a donor, we'd need his help. He agreed, but I knew that he had no intention of sleeping.

That night the phone rang only once. When I realized it wasn't Mike but a medical resident concerned about another patient, I had to push myself to maintain interest.

I awoke suddenly. It was morning. There had been no call. I reached for the phone and called the ICU. The downward slide in Robert's condition had continued. His mother and father had not gone home.

I showered, and while drying muttered to myself that the morning paper's headlines should be saying "Donor urgently required." I hoped we hadn't waited too long.

Back at the hospital I rushed down the corridor to Robert's mom and dad. They were tired but alert. They said little as they searched my face for some good news. There was none. The rest of the medical team arrived. We told the parents that we would review Robert's condition and, as agreed the previous day, if no donor had been found by five o'clock, we would contact the media.

The day passed slowly. I was at the hardware store when my pager went off: "Call switchboard, Dr. Stiller. Call switchboard." I rushed to a pay phone; the operator put me through to the ICU. "What's the problem?" I asked the nurse. There was a long pause. "Dr. Stiller, Robert just died."

"Tell the parents I will be right there," I said. I looked at my watch. It was four o'clock.

The Peters were handling their loss with courage. Mrs. Peters cried, then smiled gently.

"Could they use his eyes, Dr. Stiller?"

How generous. I wondered if I would be as noble, if I had just lost a son in this way.

We agreed to stay in touch. The Peters decided to drive home that day. I checked out of the hospital and went home.

An hour later Michael called me. He sounded exhausted. And then I remembered that no one had told him that Robert had died.

"It's five o'clock," he said. "Have you decided what to do?"

"Sorry to have to tell you, Mike. Robert died just a short time ago. Thanks for all your help." There was nothing more to say.

I went out for dinner. At seven o'clock my pager beeped. It was Michael. "I just received a call. They found a heart for Robert. How's that for luck?"

I slammed down the phone. I was shaken by anger. There had to be a better way! Medical research is increasingly advanced and communication networks have turned this planet into a village; why wasn't there some way of linking the two? One thing I knew was that the present system of searching for appropriate organ donors at the time they are needed for transplants relies too much on chance. We need better planning and better coordination.

THE POTENTIAL DONOR

Some weeks later I had a speaking engagement at the annual meeting of the London Foundation. This foundation had been established to support London's community projects and initiatives. Over the years, it has assisted many nonprofit groups financially, including our medical research at University Hospital. I was expected to report on developments in the field of organ transplants.

I hadn't planned my speech but I knew I wanted to talk about the importance of organ donation. Something is very wrong when more than 25,000 patients in North America develop kidney failure each year and less than one-half of these patients receive a transplant. (And then there is the backlog of waiting patients and those needing a second transplant.) Less than 10,000 kidneys per year are transplanted to maintain the lives of other individuals, but with 20,000 to 30,000 potential donors, perfectly good kidneys are buried within bodies that no longer need them.

I am convinced that people want to give. The question is: What stops them from giving organs that they no longer need? Is the subject too unnerving or do bureaucratic barriers prevent people from donating organs? I wondered how I could urge people to understand the power of the gift of life. For someone who has just lost a loved one, the ability to help someone else can bring incredible comfort. The tragedies of early death can be given meaning when the organs of loved ones, instead of being buried, bring an extension of life to another human being.

On the afternoon of my speaking engagement, Ann, my secretary, handed me the mail. I shuffled through it. But my mind was on my speech. Suddenly I noticed an already opened letter. I moved it to the top of the pile and began to read.

May 1, 1984

Dear Dr. Stiller,

On March 1st of this year, I phoned your office and [talked] to your secretary, who suggested that I [send] you my thoughts and ideas concerning organ donations. And after watching your program today on [television], I am further encouraged to write.

On August 28, 1982 my son Jason was struck and killed

by a motor vehicle as he was riding his bike. He would have turned 13 on September 14. Of course the anguish and grief at a time like that is such that all rational acts and thoughts are cast to the side. But as in almost all situations, time eventually [restores] you to reality and thoughts of what you could have done or should have done before and after the tragic loss. I have had many moments when I wish that some or all of Jason's organs and eyes could have been used to help people less fortunate than himself. He was always a very "giving" and unselfish boy and would not have thought twice in performing such an unselfish act had he been given the opportunity to voice his opinion. When someone is taken so quickly without any preparation, organ donation unfortunately is seldom considered. It is only when the [bereaved] are alone and a lot of the hurt is gone that the possibilities are considered.

I often wonder what I would have said if someone had called me from the hospital and asked me if I would like to authorize the transplantation of Jason's organs. On reflection, I hope I would have had the presence of mind to say yes. I was at the scene of the accident within minutes and knew by a mother's instinct that my son was dead. I accepted the reality immediately as I am a very realistic person, but the tragic loss nevertheless has left me a very changed person. Jason was my whole life. He was an only child and his father died of cancer when he was only four weeks old. I lived for my son. Everything I did I did either for Jason or with Jason in mind.

Being a law clerk, I am aware of several areas that could present problems with hospital staff calling the family after a tragic loss, but I feel that it is a possibility that is worth exploring. I have discussed the possibility with a friend of mine who lost her brother in July and she didn't hesitate to say that if the hospital had approached her or her mother, they would have given their consent.

In closing, I hope that I have perhaps opened up another avenue for you or at least given you one person's [reaction to] a very urgent situation. I somehow feel, in a very small way, that I could have gone one more step for my son but that because of "our system" Jason and I were cheated. If only I could look at another human and know that my son lives on in them and that they have had another chance at life because of Jason.

I would greatly appreciate it if you would drop me a line and let me know what you think of my suggestion. If I can no longer help my son, maybe I can help someone else.

Thank you for your time, Dr. Stiller.

Sincerely,
Mrs. S.A.

My breath caught. I looked up to see Ann standing in the doorway. She noticed my eyes fill up with tears.

"A marvelous letter, isn't it?"

"Yes," I said. "Please find this lady, Ann. I want permission to read her letter this afternoon."

Later that day the auditorium was full. My close friend Bill Brady introduced me. Bill is one of the best-known community leaders and broadcasters in the London area. People know that if they want to get something done in this city, it is important to get Bill Brady on their side. Bill may be influential but he is also a tough man to convince. I knew that if I could sway him that day, he would in turn influence many others.

At the end of my presentation, I read Jason's mother's letter. The audience became charged with emotion. I looked slowly across the room. It was a critical moment for me. It was time to push open a door onto a medical frontier fraught with difficulties but also filled with unlimited possibilities.

"The time has come," I said, "to end the cheating of countless Jasons in this country. It's time to stimulate public interest and concern, to get government, medical and legal professionals off their traditional rockers and take the luck out of organ transplantation."

I gathered up my notes, and as I walked toward the door, a

young woman with a tear-stained face held out her hand. As I acknowledged her thanks, I wondered why she was so moved.

"I'm Jason's mother," she whispered.

I clasped her hand and said nothing. Her mind must have been on Jason. I was thinking of Robert.

Something important happened to me that day. I realized with intense clarity that we needed to work hard to educate the public, as well as the medical profession, to bring about change in the system used for transplantation. Determined to ensure that the good-luck, bad-luck story of Robert was not repeated, I turned to Bill Brady, who was chairing the London Foundation meeting that day. Although I had not discussed this specifically with him, we were very close friends and we had talked of the dilemma and the matter of what appeared to be a lack of response from the public. I turned to him and said, "Bill Brady, if you will join me in this adventure, your life will be changed from this day forward."

A few days later, after much discussion, we founded Transplant International (TI) in southwestern Ontario, born not just out of urgency and need, but because of a mother's letter, a letter that caused us both to think about the terrible inequity and imbalance between need and willingness to give. Something had to be done. At that time, none of us realized that our agenda would affect so many lives, even though early in our formation the number of kidney transplants in our area increased from 28 to 58 per million.

TI's national board is made up of representatives from the medical and business communities, as well as people who have undergone a transplant. Members of the association make strong public appeals for organ donations and speak to doctors and medical associations, asking medical professionals to do all they can to inform and encourage families about to lose a loved one, to authorize an organ donation. TI has also galvanized the Canadian Medical Association to promote the signing of organ donor cards and to post this information in doctors' offices.

A BETTER MEANS OF SUPPLYING ORGANS

Today we have gone beyond simply repairing diseased or worn-out organs. Organs can now be replaced. The medical break-through that made this possible was the discovery of the drug cyclosporine in the early 1970s. Cyclosporine stops the immune system from attacking and rejecting the organ that has been transplanted. This drug has brought about a revolution in medicine. While it has some side effects, it works effectively in allowing new organs to be integrated into the recipients' bodies.

However, this medical advance is only a beginning in the field of organ transplants. Each year, we learn more about the body and how it functions in response to transplants. Medical technology is also improving.

The most serious problems hampering transplants are not medical, but logistical. A society does not move easily from one custom — seeing a body embalmed, lying in a casket and then lowered into the ground — to another, that of removing organs from the dead person and transferring them to another person's body. The societal resistance to transplants is strong. Some people feel that their loved one's body is sacred and should not be tampered with. To convince these people that there is meaning to be found in contributing organs so that another human being can go on living is not easy. What we need is an entire reorientation in terms of how people in our society think of life and death. The public must be educated about the important realities of transplants.

We look for leadership from the medical profession and from hospital administrations, but unfortunately this leadership is not always there. It takes emotional effort and precious moments out of a busy physician's schedule to help a grieving relative understand that the choice of organ donation is meaningful for all. The attending physician must then go through the administrative process of seeing to it that the organs are removed at the right time and that the medical community is informed that particular organs are available. These are enormous responsibilities.

Most hospitals still do not have an organ donation policy. They neither encourage doctors to discuss donation of organs nor provide the necessary support systems. If hospitals don't follow up by encouraging donation, all the sophisticated treatment in the world will not solve the problem of organ shortages. However, if a hospital establishes a written policy whereby its personnel are encouraged to discuss organ donation with the next of kin, we can at least be ensured that people are made aware of their options. Also, when hospital staff contribute to the writing of a policy, this endeavor heightens their own awareness of the issues as well as their sense of involvement in decision-making.

The public, too, has a vital role to play. As people come to recognize the benefit of finding meaning in the midst of tragedy, they can put pressure on their doctors, ensuring that more organs are transplanted.

The government has a responsibility to promote the availability of transplants. Increasingly, provincial governments are creating regulations to encourage donation. In most Canadian provinces and American states, for example, the government has included a form on each driver's license on which the license-holder can sign a declaration permitting a physician, in event of death, to make available some or all organs for transplant. The problems are, first, to encourage people to sign the form; second, to encourage hospital personnel to check the license to see if the donor portion has been signed; and third, to encourage people who have signed the form to inform their families, who would be asked for consent.

The cost of organ transplants is an issue confronting the medical community, insurance companies and governments. While the initial costs may be high, organ transplants are cost-effective when compared with continuous hospital care for dying patients.

Another area needing improvement was the listing of both patients waiting for an organ and organs available. The time between removing a heart from a donor and transferring it to a recipient is short. Immediate, up-to-date information about the availability of an organ is critical. Setting up and maintaining an information network is costly, but imperative.

As chief of a major transplant center, I observe, week after week, the tragedies of many Roberts who could live and regain health, if only a donor could be found. Without a donor, these patients die, remain blind or remain attached to machines. The solution lies in the love and responsiveness of people like Jason's mother. Jason in his condition could not in fact have been a heart donor; nevertheless, his mother's story points to the boundless opportunities that are blocked by inadequate communication of the facts concerning transplantation and organ donations, and by defects in our medical system in its approach to transplants.

In theory, there should be no lack of donors. As Jason's mother observed, it's not that people show no interest, but that too few families are given the opportunity to demonstrate charity when a loved one dies.

STATE OF THE ART

I AM OFTEN ASKED, "How successful *is* transplantation? Is there a good chance a patient will live after receiving an organ transplant?"

The success rate of organ transplants has risen dramatically over the past few years. Today we expect that more than 75 percent of those who receive an organ transplant will live a productive life. That percentage jumps to more than 95 percent if the transplanted tissue is taken from a brother or sister with an identical tissue type.

Too many doctors in North America continue to believe that transplantation is still experimental medicine. In fact, transplantation is a proven therapy with a far greater success rate than many other treatments offered by physicians. A patient who is diagnosed as having cancer of the stomach, kidney, bowel, esophagus, pancreas, liver or lymph nodes has a far less likelihood of surviving therapy than a patient who receives a heart transplant.

The variety of organ transplants is increasing each year. The technology is improving and research findings into how the cells work are permitting heretofore impossible organ and tissue transplants.

Kidneys are the best-known organs for transplantation as they are the most frequently performed and can come from live, as well as dead, donors. The lung transplant is one of the most difficult because the lung is so fragile; lung and heart-lung transplants are less frequently performed because only 15 to 20 percent of heart donors have lungs that are suitable for donation. The liver is the most difficult transplant, to perform surgically. The pancreas is transplanted, which may mean the entire pancreas is transplanted, a part of it or just the islets which are responsible for producing insulin. Skin transplantation is proving useful for burn victims. Corneas, bones and heart valves can be "banked" — preserved for various periods of time until needed. Also the cornea can be taken from a dead donor even though the rest of the donor's body was not useable because of age or disease. The bone transplant is used for a variety of bone reconstructions in the recipient's body. Bone marrow, taken from a living donor, may be transplanted, usually for treatment of leukemia.

The most experimental transplants today are partial liver transplants taken from a live donor and the small bowel transplant. First trials of the former are only just beginning and will require rigorous evaluation.

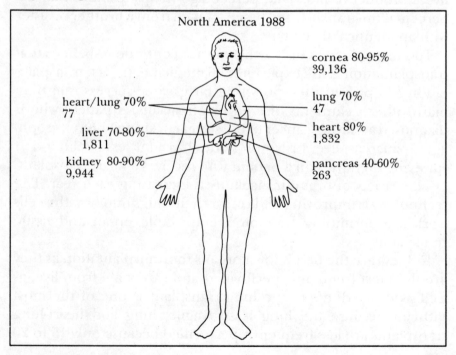

North America 1988

cornea 80-95%
39,136

heart/lung 70%
77

lung 70%
47

liver 70-80%
1,811

heart 80%
1,832

kidney 80-90%
9,944

pancreas 40-60%
263

The dramatic improvement in the success rate for transplants is due largely to the use of cyclosporine, a drug sometimes called the "penicillin of transplants." Before the discovery of cyclosporine the success rate for kidney transplants was 45 to 50 percent. When cyclosporine was introduced in 1978, the success rate jumped to 80 percent. By 1978, heart transplants had almost ceased (except at Stanford University in California). While surgeons could successfully transfer a heart from a donor to a recipient, in only 45 percent of transplants would the recipient's body accept the new organ. Medical science's failure to ensure that the recipient's body would accept the new heart led to an increased reluctance on the part of medical centers to engage in heart transplants. With the introduction of cyclosporine, the success rate shot up to 80 percent. Liver transplants, performed mostly by Dr. Tom Starzl, who worked in Denver, Colorado, and is now at the University of Pittsburgh, surged from a survival rate of only 35 percent to an amazing 75 percent. And heart-lung transplants, once considered an extraordinary risk, were initiated at Stanford University; at University Hospital in London, Ontario; and at a number of other centers. With the help of cyclosporine, heart-lung transplants achieved a 60 percent success rate.

From time to time, major breakthroughs in medicine change the course of certain diseases and save the lives of millions of people. The discovery of penicillin in 1928 by Dr. Alexander Fleming was one such breakthrough. The discovery of insulin by Dr. Frederick Banting and Dr. Charles Best in 1922 was another. Today Drs. Calne, White and Borel have surmounted the obstacle of organ rejection by means of cyclosporine.

TRANSPLANTATION AND THE IMMUNE SYSTEM

The body's rejection of a new organ is normal; the same defense system that protects us from infection also rejects a new organ.

The immune response is one of the most fascinating systems

that nature has devised for the maintenance of life. The integrity of the body throughout life is controlled by this system. Every day, whether we're sitting in a crowded bus, working in an office or watching television at home, we are surrounded by viruses, bacteria and fungi. It rarely occurs to us that as we interact with others we might contract a serious infection. We expect our body's immune system to sort out what will and will not harm us. But in order for the immune system to do that, it has to be able to distinguish a foreign "invader" from what is "self."

The idea of "self" is determined in our mother's uterus at a very early stage in our development. The bone marrow produces three key cells that shape the immune response. The immune response is an orchestrated system responsible for preventing the invasion and destruction of the body's cells.

Think of the immune system as an army. In this analogy, the *macrophage cells,* produced by the bone marrow, are the scouts. They are also the army's cleanup crew. They identify any "trespasser" in the body, carry a piece of that invader to the army's "general," and then receive instructions as to whether an attack should be launched.

The general is known as the T-helper cell. Although this cell originates in the bone marrow or liver of the fetus while it is still in the uterus, it develops in the thymus, a gland located in the lower neck. It is here that the cell "learns" about all of the tissues of the body and this knowledge of self is locked in its "memory" forever.

The third type of cell is called the B-cell, which produces antibodies and functions as the "artillery" of the immune system.

"Self" is a very precise system, which can be demonstrated in an experiment on a pregnant white rat, close to term. The rat is anesthetized. Its uterus is opened up and one of the nine pups is removed while it is still attached to the umbilical cord. Skin from a black rat is grafted onto the skin of this white pup. The pup is returned to its mother's uterus, which is sewn up. The mother rat wakes up and, at full term, delivers her pups.

When the pups are mature, skin is taken from the same black

rat that served as the donor above and is then transplanted as a surface patch onto the skin of all the white pups. Eight pups will reject the transplanted skin from the black rat because it is not self. The ninth will accept the transplant. Why? Because while the one pup was still in its mother's uterus, the original skin graft from the black rat was interpreted as self and became locked into the memory of this pup's T-helper cell.

Ironically, we must override the body's immune system in order to ensure a successful organ transplant from one individual to another. When a heart is placed in the chest of a recipient, the macrophages (the scouts or scavengers) pick up a piece of the new heart and present it to the T-helper cell (the general). Recognizing a foreign invader, the T-helper cell sends out a message to launch an attack. This message is given to cousins of the T-helper cell, who become "killer-cells" and attack the transplanted heart. At the general's command, the B-cells (the artillery) manufacture antibodies to launch at the new heart; the antibodies eventually close off the blood vessels. This process of rejection takes about 96 hours. Then the scavengers move in. Within seven to ten days, the organ is rejected and destroyed.

Remember the first heart transplant, performed in 1967 by Dr. Christiaan Barnard in South Africa? Barnard left the operating room and announced his successful heart transplant to the press. While an excited world held its breath, the heart recipient showed improvement on the second day. By day three, he was apparently coming off the critical list. By the fourth day (96 hours following the transplant), fever had been noted — the scout was presenting the foreign tissue to the general and the general was sending out his first signal. This signal produced the fever. The patient got worse. Inflammation set in. Death occurred within three weeks of the transplant.

The heart recipient's body was simply doing what is was supposed to do: it was ridding itself of something that wasn't self. The key to successful transplants lay not in making the important surgical connections (although, without successful and skilled surgery, transplantation is only a theory), but rather in controlling the immune response in such a way that rejection would not occur.

In the early days of transplant research, the agents used to control the immune response were largely derived from anticancer agents. Although this approach worked, it worked too well. In fact, the immune response was generally destroyed and these agents made the whole body sick. Such an approach is equivalent to trying to repel an enemy's advancing army by spraying the whole country with a poison: not only is the advancing army affected but citizens also get sick. When we used drugs from anticancer agents, not only were the T-helper cells and the macrophages affected, but also normal body cells were attacked. The patient would then die of infection, cancer or general toxicity.

Prior to the use of cyclosporine, transplants were experimental, just as the treatment of infection was experimental prior to the discovery of penicillin. But the treatment for rejection was often so inexact that frequently one of two situations occurred. The organ sometimes survived, but the patient died of infection. Alternatively, if the patient managed to resist infection, the organ was rejected. The solution lay, obviously, in finding a way to control rejection without stripping the body of its defenses.

THE DISCOVERY OF CYCLOSPORINE

Just as penicillin resulted by chance, from a fungus found growing in a petri dish, so did cyclosporine. In 1970, a brilliant discovery changed the science of transplants. Sandoz Corporation, a large multinational pharmaceutical company based in Basel, Switzerland, had directed its executives, scientists and sales representatives to take plastic bags with them wherever they travelled. Whenever they arrived at a new place they were to scoop up some dirt from the ground, put it in the plastic bag, seal the bag and label it with the location. Upon returning home, they would take the sealed bags to the research center. Samples of earth were placed in a petri dish and cultured. Why? The company was looking for new antibiotics, just as Fleming had been when he grew a mold and found penicillin.

The Sandoz research strategy worked. Scientists discovered that a sample from a northwestern fjord in Norway and one from Minnesota contained the same fungus. (No one has been able to say why the same fungus was found in these two locations. Maybe a Norwegian carried it to Minnesota on the heel of his boot!) The fungus produced an interesting substance which was far from a spectacular antibiotic, however. In fact, its characteristics made it a poor antibiotic; it seemed to do the opposite of what an antibiotic was supposed to do. Researchers found that this new agent affected a test animal's immune system, but it made the animal *more* susceptible to infection. Sandoz decided the fungus did not justify further study and halted all research on it.

One man did not follow orders. A brilliant Swiss scientist, Dr. Jean François Borel, was working in one of the Sandoz Corporation laboratories, screening for new agents. He observed that the unusual new agent, which he called "cyclosporine," seemed to affect the T-helper cell in a very specific way. He later described his findings to the scientific world, pointing out cyclosporine's potential benefits for organ transplantation.

How does cyclosporine work? Just as penicillin kills bacteria without injuring the patient, cyclosporine controls the cells that cause rejection, without harming the rest of the body. To extend the previous analogy, it acts like a sleeping pill administered to the army general (the T-helper cell) and it affects only the T-helper cell. When a patient takes cyclosporine, it's as though the general falls asleep. Even though the scout (macrophage cell) presents the T-helper cell with pieces of the invading organ, no command is issued; no killer-cells are generated; no antibodies (artillery) are launched; and the patient lives in peaceful coexistence with the transplanted foreign organ.

When Professor Borel first discovered cyclosporine's effect

upon the immune system, his interest was purely scientific. He was intrigued by its ability to target the T-helper cell. It wasn't long before he realized that cyclosporine might be used to inhibit or suppress the immune response in the human body, thus enabling the transplanted organ to survive.

Borel set out to test his hypothesis by injecting both red blood cells from sheep as well as cyclosporine into the body of a mouse. To his delight, the animal did not produce antibodies. He next performed a skin transplant upon the mouse. He demonstrated that when the mouse received cyclosporine, the animal lost its ability to reject the skin, as would normally be the case.

Although the effects of cyclosporine were not publicized until two or three years later, these early studies pointed the way for scientists, physicians and surgeons. Professor Borel's work inspired Sir Roy Calne of Cambridge University and his associate, Professor David White, to do further testing in both rats and dogs, after which they concluded that successful transplantation could indeed take place with the help of cyclosporine.

When Sir Roy Calne described the potency of the new drug to the world medical community, there was a rush to get samples to test in other studies. At the International Transplant Congress held in Rome in 1978, the most sought-after consultant was Professor Borel. Many scientists requested his permission to allow the drug to be used for research. Nevertheless, he resisted most of these requests because cyclosporine was an unproven entity; the toxicity of the drug had not been established. It wasn't until the early 1980s that cyclosporine's full effect was understood.

I tried to arrange an interview with Professor Borel at the Rome conference in 1978, but without success. Then, following a papal audience in St. Peter's Square, I looked for a taxi to escape the pouring rain. I managed to commandeer one for the ride back to the Hotel Caballero Hilton. I noticed Professor Borel trying to hail a cab and invited him to join me. As soon as the taxi door had closed behind him, I asked, "Now can we talk about how I can get this cyclosporine?"

THE WONDER OF CYCLOSPORINE

Since 1978, cyclosporine has dominated our clinical interests. It has allowed us to begin to fulfill the dream of transplanting any organ, including the intestine and entire limbs, both in the laboratory and in the hospital. Today, with the aid of cyclosporine and other anti-rejection drugs, three-quarters of all transplant patients can expect to experience a restoration of life.

Cyclosporine is administered to patients orally twice a day either in a capsule or liquid form. As long as the patient takes it as prescribed, the rejection factor is greatly diminished.

Ideally, patients receive cyclosporine before the organ is transplanted. The earlier it is administered, the better. If the T-helper cells are sedated by the cyclosporine and put into a resting phase before transplant surgery, then rejection can be completely averted. The drug must then be taken for life, once or twice a day.

It is important to monitor the dosages of cyclosporine carefully; it can become toxic if given in too large a dose. Because cyclosporine inhibits the defense mechanism that is activated by the immune system to protect the body, there is a possibility of infection if too much of the drug is used. Even when appropriate doses are given, the incidence of cancer in the transplant patient is increased compared with the normal population. The most serious side effect is on kidney functioning, which must be carefully monitored.

A bothersome but not critical side effect of cyclosporine is a cosmetic one. The drug stimulates the growth of hair, sometimes producing a "Brooke Shields" eyebrow or generating hair growth on a man's bald pate. It may also cause hair to grow on the arms and legs of both women and men. Also, some patients receiving large doses experience an increased growth rate in the gums.

PERFORMING A HEART TRANSPLANT

Today, hundreds of hospitals in North America perform transplants, and the number of transplants is increasing every month. At present, successful transplants can be done on the heart, lungs, liver, kidneys, pancreas, cornea, skin, bone marrow, bone and intestine.

Orchestrating a transplant begins by first identifying a patient who would benefit from receiving a new organ. This must be done as early as possible so that organ failure does not cause the patient's body to deteriorate.

In this brief overview of one type of organ transplant — the heart transplant — I'll use the example of a patient with a defective heart to explain how transplantation actually takes place. Transplanting other major organs works in essentially the same way as does a heart transplant. One major difference is that in the transplant of organs such as the kidney or liver, the heart-lung machine is not used.

When the patient is brought into hospital, all the recipient's body systems are checked, so that the medical team has a comprehensive assessment of the patient's total condition. In the case of a patient with a defective heart, we check to ensure that the lungs, kidneys and intestine are healthy and that there is no infection that could endanger the new heart, once it is implanted.

As soon as the surgeon is notified that a donor heart is available, the selected patient is prepared for the operating room (OR). Just like when a patient is about to receive a blood transfusion, the blood groups of the donor and the recipient will have been matched. If the donor's blood group is O, then the donor heart can go to any recipient, regardless of blood group. But if the donor's blood group is A, then the donor heart can go only to a recipient whose blood group is also A. The same is true if the donor's blood group is B or AB.

The size and weight of both the donor and the recipient are checked, especially with extra-renal transplants. This is important for two reasons. First, when replacing a heart with another heart, a surgeon has to reconnect the blood vessels, and this is more difficult if the donor heart is much smaller than the recipient's heart. Also the size of the chest cavity of both donor and recipient is important in heart transplants. It is difficult to put a large donor heart into the chest cavity of a small recipient.

Tissue typing and cross-matching are also important, but more so for kidneys. (Often there is not time before a heart or liver transplant to determine tissue type.) The white blood cells are obtained from the donor's spleen or blood or lymph nodes and compared with blood serum from the recipient. The closer the match, the better the recipient's chances of accepting the new organ. The recipient is also checked for antibodies in the blood against the donor in the cross-match test.

When all the checking and tests have been done, two teams — the retrieval team and the transplant team — go to work.

The retrieval team consists of a surgeon and a transplant coordinator or technician. They travel to the hospital where the donor is being maintained. When they arrive, the donor is taken to the operating room. No anesthetic is necessary when the donor's heart is removed because the donor's brain is dead. However, an anesthetist monitors the donor's blood pressure.

The area around the heart is prepared so that cutting and tying the blood vessels and removing the organ can be done within two to five minutes. Speed is now of the essence.

Before the surgeon removes the heart, large volumes of cold fluid are run through it. The vessels are then clamped and cut. The surgeon removes the heart and repeats the perfusing so that the heart is free of blood. The organ is packaged for transportation to the recipient's hospital.

While the donor is being operated on, the transplant team begins its work. The recipient is taken to the operating room and given a general anesthetic. The transplant surgeon waits for the retrieval surgeon to call, indicating that the heart has been obtained, detailing the condition of the organ and giving the transplant surgeon the go-ahead to start removing the diseased heart from the recipient. The recipient's chest is opened and the breast bone is split. The patient is put on a heart-lung bypass machine.

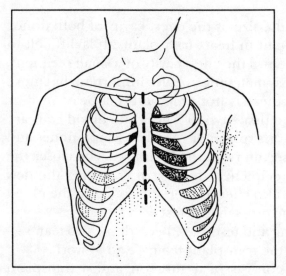

Heart transplant. Incision line in recipient for heart transplant.

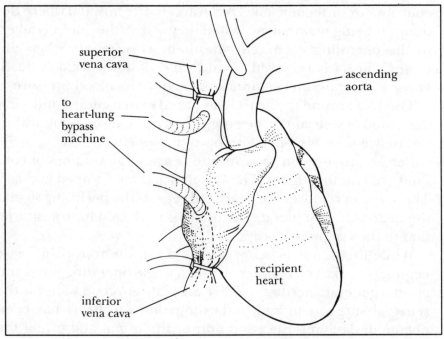

superior
vena cava

ascending
aorta

to
heart-lung
bypass
machine

recipient
heart

inferior
vena cava

The recipient is placed on a heart-lung bypass machine before the diseased heart is removed. Tubes are inserted into the recipient's superior and inferior venae cavae (veins that receive blood from the upper and lower parts of the body, respectively, and return it to the heart).

The heart-lung bypass machine operates as the heart and lungs for the patient. Tubes are inserted into the recipient's superior and inferior venae cavae (veins that receive blood from the upper and lower body and return it to the heart). These tubes take the blood from the body to the heart-lung machine, which acts as an artificial lung putting oxygen back into the blood. The blood is returned by an arterial line into the aorta. The aorta has been clamped so the blood is diverted into the body.

The area surrounding the recipient's heart is dissected and bands are placed around the blood vessels to be cut. The transplant surgeon then waits for the retrieval surgeon to arrive with the new heart.

The donor heart is taken from a plastic bag containing cold fluid. The transplant surgeon examines the heart to determine that it is in good condition and that it will sustain the stress of transplantation. The length and size of the new heart's vessels are measured so that the surgeon knows how much vessel length to leave when he removes the old heart.

Within minutes the recipient's vessels are clamped and cut and the old heart is taken out, leaving an empty cavity. The new heart is taken from the cold solution, its vessels are trimmed to match the recipient's vessels, and a continuous line of sutures join the left atria of donor and recipient.

In order to make the procedure easier, part of the right and left atria of the old heart is kept in place within the recipient. This cuts down on the number of veins to be sutured when the new heart is inserted.

The heart has been joined at the left and right atria, then at the aorta and pulmonary artery. (See the diagrams.) A little blood is allowed to enter the new heart, a needle is inserted through the upper part of the heart wall and the air trapped inside is sucked out. When no more air can be obtained and when suturing has stopped any leaks at the junctions of the vessels, the vessels are unclamped and the new heart begins to warm up as blood flows through it. The heart quivers and may even begin to beat on its own. If the new heart doesn't start to beat regularly but continues to quiver, electric paddles are placed on it and an electric shock is administered. The electrocardiogram shows when the donor heart has started to take over.

When the heart appears to be functioning normally, blood pressure is also normal, the patient is pink and the kidneys are putting out urine (a sign of adequate blood flowing through the organs), the tubes to the heart-lung machine are removed, the envelope around the heart is closed, the clamps holding the chest open are removed, and wire sutures are used to fit the split breastbone snugly back together. A tube is placed through an incision in the skin just below the heart so that any bleeding can be drained. The skin is then closed.

In the intensive care unit, the patient functions completely on the new heart. Except for having undergone major surgery, the patient is now healthy. Because the cause of the illness has been completely removed (and, in many cases, because the patient has received a younger organ), the heart can now provide the body

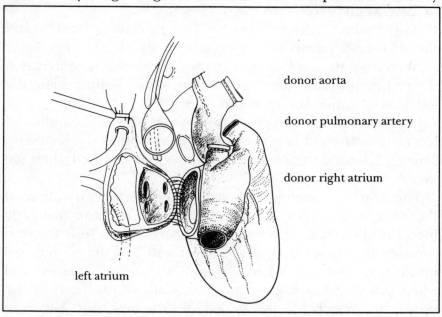

As a heart transplant begins, the donor heart's left atrium is joined with the recipient's.

with the blood flow necessary for healing. Of course, we still have rejection to treat and prevent. But for the moment health has been restored.

PERFORMING A KIDNEY TRANSPLANT

While the essential transplant procedure is the same for most organs, there are some differences. This can be seen in walking through the steps of a kidney transplant.

For a multi-organ donor, the surgeon will first flush out the organs by means of a catheter in the main artery (aorta) and then remove the organs after they are cold.

Once a kidney is removed it is placed in a basin full of saline (a salt solution) and ice. A catheter is put in the kidney's renal artery and a cold solution is run through the organ until all of the old blood in the kidney is completely removed.

The kidney is then put into a plastic bag filled with an ice-cold preservative solution. That bag is put into a sterile plastic bag to protect the kidney from contamination. Finally, the kidney is put into a cooler (literally, a picnic cooler) filled with ice-cold slush. The cooler is closed and carried to the hospital where the recipient is being prepared. The solution is kept at 4°C; if it gets much colder, it could freeze. It must be kept cold, however, to prevent metabolism and death.

For organs such as the liver, lungs, heart, kidneys and pancreas, time, and therefore the transportation factor, is critical, a matter of hours only. For the liver, the transplant time limit is 24 hours; for the heart, four to six hours; for kidneys, 24 to 48 hours; for the pancreas, 16 to 24 hours; and for lungs, less than three hours.

The donor coordinator carries the cooler into the operating room where the recipient has been prepared. The surgeon carefully removes the donor kidney from the plastic bag with forceps, trims away fat and cuts the angles of the blood vessels so that they will fit the vessels of the recipient. An incision is made

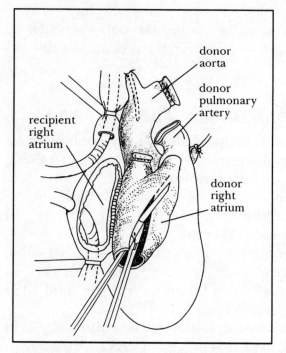

The right atrium is cut so that the circumference is approximately the size of the recipient's right atrium.

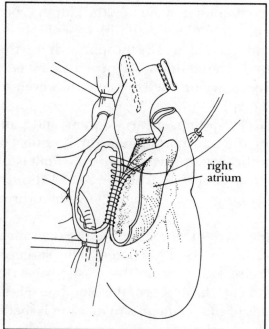

The right atria of the donor and the recipient are joined with a continuous suture.

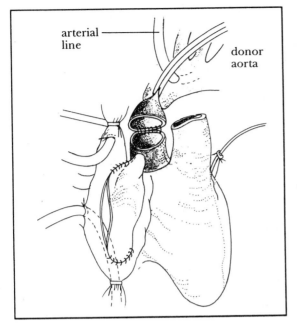

The donor aorta has been shortened for suturing to the recipient's aorta.

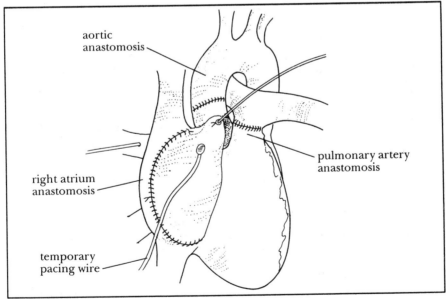

The pulmonary artery is attached to the new heart. A temporary pacing wire is often attached to the right atrium or right ventricle for the first few days following a transplant, in case the heartbeat becomes irregular.

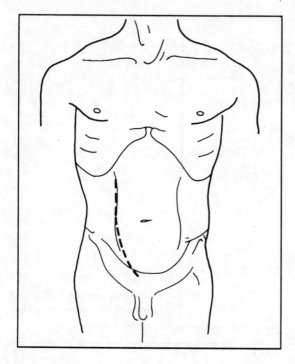

In a kidney tranplant, a curved incision line is made.

in the recipient's groin where the new kidney is to be placed.

The vessels used to hook up the new kidney are the ones that normally supply blood only to the legs. When positioned within the recipient's groin, the kidney is gently twisted around to ensure that when the vessels are sewn in place they won't kink and thus impede blood flow.

The surgeon then removes the donor kidney from the groin and puts it back in the cold solution to keep it cold while the recipient is prepared. The kidney is then placed in the recipient's body and the vessels of the donor organ are sutured to the vessels of the recipient. A special suture is used, one so fine it is difficult to see with the unaided eye.

When transplanting a kidney, the surgeon first sutures the vein and checks to make sure there are no leaks. Then the artery is sutured and checked for leaks also. Once the surgeon is sure the veins and arteries are properly sewn together, the clamps are

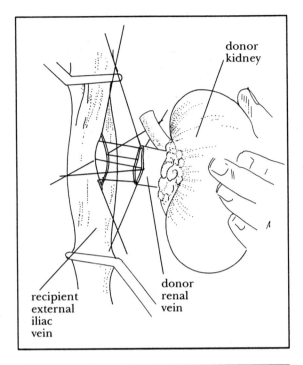

recipient external iliac vic vein

donor kidney

donor renal vein

Sutures are passed through the donor renal vein to the external iliac vein.

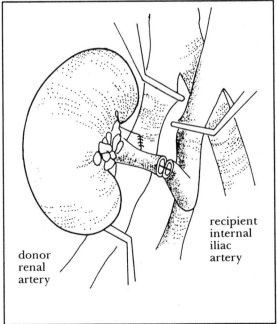

donor renal artery

recipient internal iliac artery

The renal artery is joined to the recipient's internal iliac artery or the external iliac artery.

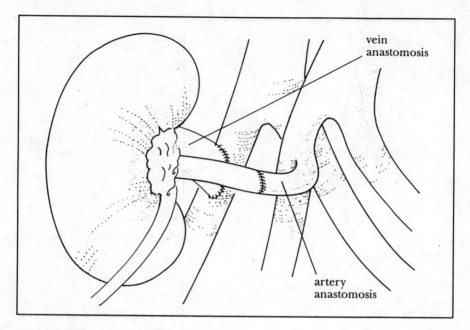

Completed kidney transplant.

removed and the kidney becomes filled with blood.

Then the surgeon deals with the ureter, which carries the urine from the kidney to the bladder. If the ureter is functioning properly, the end of the ureter is cut to the right length to fit inside the bladder. If the surgeon is satisfied that all is well, a tunnel is cut into the bladder and the lining of the ureter is sewn to the lining of the bladder.

During a kidney transplant, the old kidneys are left in the recipient and their ureters are not used. The reason for this is that there is a greater likelihood of leaks occurring if the recipient's ureter (the link between the kidney and the bladder) is used instead of the donor's ureter.

The operations just described are but two of the many kinds of transplants possible today. The diagrams show surgical procedures for other organ transplants, including multi-organ re-

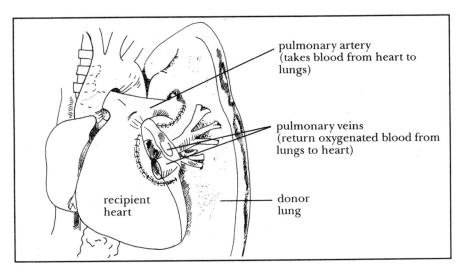

Single lung transplant. The donor's left atrium (containing the pulmonary veins), pulmonary artery and bronchial tubes are joined with the recipient's. A cardiopulmonary bypass (heart-lung) machine may be needed with a single lung transplant, but is always used for a double lung transplant. In a double lung transplant, the trachea (windpipe) is attached before the left atrium and pulmonary artery.

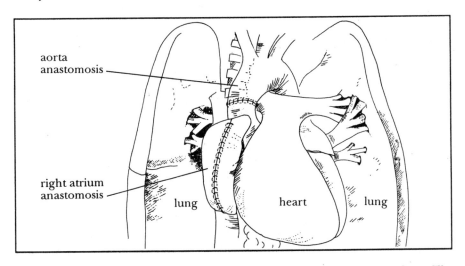

Heart-lung transplant. The patient is placed on a heart-lung bypass machine. The diseased heart and lungs are removed separately, beginning with the heart, and then the left and right lungs. The donor's trachea (windpipe), aorta and right atrium are joined with the recipient's.

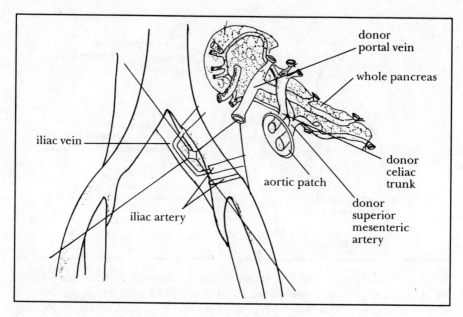

Pancreas transplant. The donor portal vein is attached to the iliac vein and the aortic patch is joined to the iliac artery.

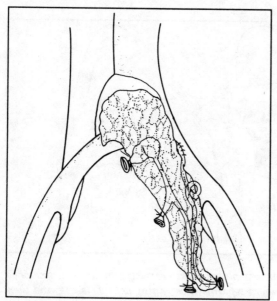

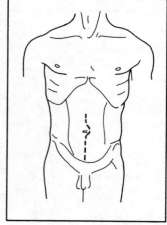

In a pancreas transplant, a lower midline incision is made.

Completed whole pancreas transplant.

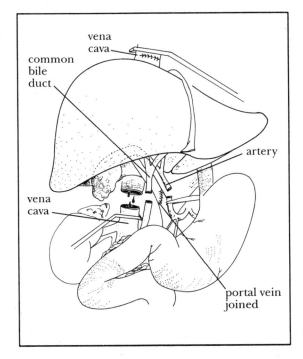

vena cava

common bile duct

vena cava

artery

portal vein joined

Liver transplant. The first attachment is between the recipient's and the donor's venae cavae above the liver. Then the donor portal vein is attached to the recipient's portal vein. Preservative solution is flushed out of the liver via the vena cava at the bottom of the liver before the donor's and recipient's venae cavae are joined, followed by the artery and common bile duct.

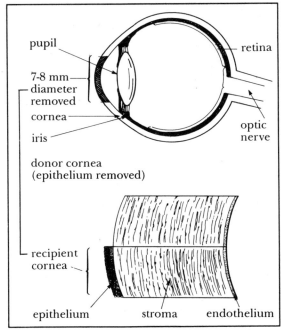

pupil

retina

7-8 mm diameter removed

cornea

iris

optic nerve

donor cornea (epithelium removed)

recipient cornea

epithelium   stroma   endothelium

Profile of the eye. In a cornea transplant, 7 to 8 mm of cornea are removed and replaced with donor cornea tissue. There are two basic types of cornea transplant: lamellar ("partial-thickness") for surface disease in the cornea; and penetrating ("full-thickness"). The majority of cornea transplants are full-thickness. The corneal suture is left in place for 12 to 14 months and is then removed as an office procedure.

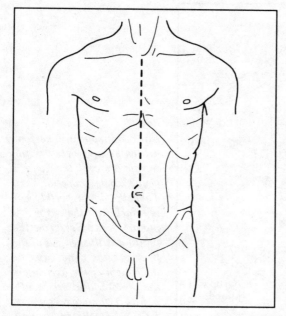

The incision for multiple organ donation extends from above the breast bone to the genital area.

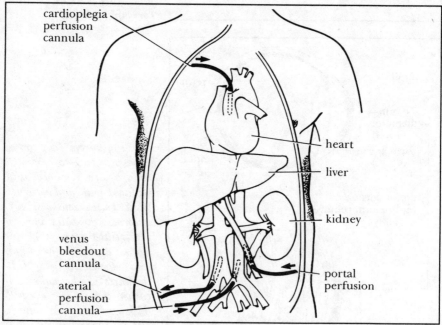

cardioplegia perfusion cannula

heart

liver

kidney

venus bleedout cannula

aterial perfusion cannula

portal perfusion

Multi-organ donor. Perfusion tubes are inserted so the organs can be flushed with a cold preservative solution before removal.

moval. As our technical skills improve, medical science will one day be able to transplant any organ. Currently, a donor can give lungs, a heart, a liver, a pancreas, eyes, skin, several bones and, in some very select transplant centers, the intestine.

Years from now we will look back in astonishment at the medical advances made in the early 1980s. We will recognize and commemorate the contributions of pioneers such as Sir Peter Medawar, a British immunologist who received the Nobel Prize for his work on the immune system and who is known as the father of transplantation science; Jean François Borel; Roy Calne; Tom Starzl; Paul Terasaki and many others, all part of a dedicated group who propelled the medical world into the 21st century.

THE SUCCESSFUL TRANSPLANT

WHAT HAPPENS WHEN a person receives a new organ? What physical and emotional traumas must be faced while undergoing transplant procedures? What emotional traumas must a bereaved family deal with before making an organ donation? These questions are best answered by looking at actual, successful transplants.

FROM A RECIPIENT'S POINT OF VIEW

March, 1985. A nagging cough following a trip to Hawaii seemed a small price to pay for a wonderful holiday. But after numerous medications for colds and bronchitis failed, the cough persisted. So Fred Casswell from Regina, Saskatchewan made an appointment with his family doctor in late April.

A 42-year-old high school teacher, Fred had always enjoyed good health. But he was slightly worried when his doctor called him in for an x-ray in June and then, two days later, asked him to return.

The diagnosis? Fred's heart was enlarged. His heart was seriously diseased and, according to the cardiologist, there was little chance it would ever improve. "As a matter of fact," the doctor commented, "somewhere down the road, you might need a heart transplant."

Fred's reaction was disbelief: "This guy has to be kidding. A transplant? He can't be serious." But after talking with his wife Carol, Fred recognized the need to stop panicking and instead plan rationally for the future.

The cardiologist prescribed medication and complete rest, but Fred's condition didn't improve. Then he felt another cold coming on in September. It wasn't long before both he and Carol knew his illness was more than a cold.

"It was an awful period," recalled Fred. "Carol would stay awake at night, unknown to me, to watch over me. Sometimes I'd stop breathing and she would nudge me awake enough so I would begin to breathe again. It was incomprehensible to Carol that someone she had known only in perfect health was wasting away before her eyes. Yet she did not show fear and gave me all the support I needed."

On November 7, 1985, Fred was admitted to Regina Pasqua Hospital. "I lay there wondering what was going to happen to me. It suddenly dawned on me that exactly 22 years ago, to the day, my dad had died of heart failure at the age of 53."

The cardiologist in Regina contacted our transplant unit in London. We agreed that Fred's condition was serious enough to warrant a heart transplant and we suggested he be moved to London where we could examine him more thoroughly. And so, on December 10, Fred, Carol and their mothers flew from Regina to London.

"I think every intern took my case history," Fred recollected. "Dr. Bill Kostuk, the attending cardiologist in London, came into my room, pulled the flimsy white curtains around my bed, and in words meant only for Carol's and my ears told us my heart was in very bad shape. The only option was a transplant. When I asked for his projection regarding how long I could live with my old heart, he replied that, while there was no way he could predict, he thought about six months, at best.

One day a patient in a blue track suit, beads of sweat trickling down his face from exercise, walked into Fred's room. He introduced himself as Peter Chabaniuk. Fred was flabbergasted to learn that Peter had had a heart transplant just four weeks earlier! Needless to say, meeting Peter was extremely encouraging for Fred.

Fred and Carol now began the agonizing wait for a suitable donor heart. They sublet the home of a London family near the University Hospital. After 17 days, Fred learned that a heart had been found. Fred had already been prepared for the surgery and he and Carol were waiting for a call from the operating room when they learned that the heart had been judged unsuitable. "Don't worry about it, Fred," Carol comforted her husband. "We'll just look at this as a dress rehearsal for the right one." The wait continued . . .

January 26, 1986. 9:30 AM. That morning, Fred had been at the hospital's outpatient department for a checkup. We had equipped him with a pocket pager so that the transplant recipient coordinator could contact him at any moment. He left with his beeper and returned to the house.

11:55 AM. Michael Bloch, the senior transplant donor coordinator, received a call from a hospital in the Maritimes, where a 19-year-old man had died. Although brain death had not been declared, the man appeared to be clinically dead. Brain tracing by means of an electroencephalograph would be done later that evening.

January 27, 11:30 AM. The young man had been declared brain-dead. Michael spoke to Dr. McKenzie about whether or not the donor heart would be suitable for Fred. They both agreed it would be.

Connie Santamaria, the transplant recipient coordinator, contacted the switchboard and had them beep Fred on his pocket pager. Fred returned the call within minutes, and was summoned to see Dr. McKenzie.

"Fred," said Dr. McKenzie, "it looks as if we have a heart for you." This was no longer a dress rehearsal. The Casswells remembered their earlier experience, when they had learned at the last moment that the potential donor heart wasn't suitable. But with the news of another heart they both began to feel excited.

Michael was on the phone arranging for a jet to pick up the retrieval team in London at five o'clock that afternoon, fly them to the east coast, pick up the donor heart and return to London that night.

London, 5:01 PM. The plane carrying the retrieval team departed from the airport in London.

En route, 5:21 PM. Michael called the operating room in the donor's city and spoke with Dr. Owen Audain, the surgeon in charge, who was instructed to prepare the donor for organ removal. Although brain-dead, the young man was still on life-support systems to prolong the life of his other organs.

Donor's city, 6:49 PM. The retrieval team from London, including Michael, arrived at the Moncton hospital. After scrubbing, Dr. McKenzie made the chest incision and spread the ribs.

8:45 PM. Michael called the University Hospital in London and instructed the on-duty physician, Dr. Nader Tadros, to prepare Fred for surgery, because it appeared that the donor heart was healthy. Michael said they hoped to have the heart removed from the donor within the next half hour. He estimated they would be back in London by 11 o'clock that night.

9:13 PM. A tube was inserted into the aorta in preparation to flush the heart with preservation solution. The aorta was clamped to force the solution through the heart so it was flushed clean of blood and cooled. The heart quickly lost its reddish-pink color as the donor's blood was flushed out. The heartbeat slowed and in a matter of seconds stopped. The heart was removed, cleaned and placed in a bag containing a cold solution.

London, 9:30 PM. After saying "see you a little later" to Carol, Fred was taken to the operating room and put under anesthetic. His chest was sterilized and he was draped with operating sheets. But no incision was made. The surgeon was waiting for a call from the retrieval team to say they had boarded the plane and were flying back to London.

Donor's city, 9:40 PM. Dr. McKenzie and Michael Bloch boarded the plane for their return trip to London.

En route, 10:00 PM. Aboard the jet, Dr. McKenzie called the operating room at the London hospital to say that all was well and that the transplant team could begin to operate on Fred.

London, 10:20 PM. Fred's chest cavity was opened and he was put on a heart-lung bypass machine so that his body could function during the transplant operation.

While Fred was lying in the operating room, Carol phoned some family and friends in Regina to update them and then sat with her mother and Fred's mother in a small room at the hospital. Carol looked out the window, hoping to see the plane transporting Fred's new heart.

London, 11:48 PM. Dr. McKenzie and his team entered the operating room in London and announced that the heart was viable and ready for transplant.

London, January 28, 12:25 AM. Dr. McKenzie had scrubbed and began to remove the damaged heart.

12:35 AM. Fred's damaged heart was removed. The new donor heart was taken from the storage bag. Its vessels were trimmed to match Fred's aorta and pulmonary artery and the left and right atria were trimmed to receive the patch of atria that had been left in Fred's chest cavity. The heart from the young man who had died a few hours earlier was sutured into Fred's body. The new heart was ready to begin pumping 180 L of blood an hour; with the surging blood would come new life for Fred.

The first words Fred heard when he regained consciousness were Carol's: "Fred, it's over! You did it!" But most of all he remembers the incredible sensation of rebirth. "Dr. Stiller," he said, "having this new heart is like walking into a dark room and having someone turn on a lightswitch so you can see again."

Recovery from a transplant operation is not pleasant. Machines in the intensive care unit constantly whirr and buzz. It seems that every few minutes, someone is poking or prodding some part of your body. In Fred's words: "I remember lying in bed and I couldn't get to sleep. I heard this funny noise. It was kind of like an ocean wave pounding on a shore. Whoosh, whoosh, whoosh! What is that? I wondered. I kept thinking it was the monitor, but there was no monitor. All of a sudden, it struck me: it was my heart. Incredible! It may sound strange, but I began talking to my heart. I said, 'You're doing a great job in there. Don't quit. Just keep it up.'"

The medical staff's primary postoperative goal is to stabilize the patient and to make sure that the antirejection drug is adequate. This is usually accomplished within 12 hours.

The second goal is to remove from the patient, as soon as possible, all intrusive instruments used in the operation, such as respiratory tubes, drains and catheters.

After allowing the wound to heal for 72 to 96 hours, mobilization of the patient begins. As soon as possible, patients are encouraged to become active. In our transplant unit, we have a room equipped with exercise bicycles. Our aim is to reorient the patient towards health and to offset preoccupation with sickness.

During this critical postoperative phase, the team is acutely aware of the possibility of organ rejection, infection and drug toxicity. The nurses, surgeon and recipient coordinator all cast a wary eye over the temperature chart, anxiously monitoring the trend, and scrutinize any tests that might indicate rejection. In the case of a kidney transplant, any increase in the patient's weight over the previous day is monitored. Increasing blood flow through the kidney is a good sign that the newly transplanted kidney is working.

In the case of a heart transplant, some early signs of rejection are fever, shortness of breath and weight gain. To determine if rejection is occurring, a catheter is slipped through a vein into the heart and a small piece of the heart is removed and examined under a microscope. The doctor watches closely for irregularity in the heartbeat, an increase of fluid on the lungs or an increase in the size of the heart.

A lung transplant is judged to be successful on the basis of the lung's ability to oxygenate the blood. The amount of oxygen in the blood is measured at regular intervals. A chest x-ray is critical. Sometimes just listening to the chest can indicate rejection. As with a new heart, a biopsy is critical. A doctor always regards signs of rejection with caution, as an infection could be mimicking rejection in the patient.

Recovery time varies with each patient. Fred Casswell was exhilarated after surgery. The pain of healing wounds cooled his heels for the first few days. But within three days, Fred was up and walking.

Fred's rapid recovery is not unusual. What surprises most visitors upon seeing someone who has just had a transplant, is how wonderful the person looks. The simple fact is that the organ that had made the recipient an invalid is now gone. And in its place is a healthy, fully functioning organ that can rejuvenate the entire body.

Most major transplant operations do not require a long post-operative recovery period, as long as the body does not reject the new organ and no infection develops. If the new organ is accepted by the body and the rest of the patient's organs function normally, the only real problem is the healing of the tissue where the new organ was attached and where the incision was made. In the case of a heart or lung transplant, because the rib cage has been stretched open, its healing is a vital part of recovery.

For Fred, the realization that his physical well-being was at the expense of someone else's life was most sobering. "I realized I was here and someone else had died. I thought of what [the donor's] family had gone through. I cried for his family and I cried for my family. I thought about what it meant to be alive, that by the process of organ donation — this miracle — I had been given the gift of life."

While Fred was recovering, he struck up a friendship with a young priest, Father Rick Janisse, one of our hospital's chaplains.

One day they discussed the death of Mike, a 21-year-old, whose transplant surgery had failed. Fred asked Father Rick why a 21-year-old had died while he, a 42-year-old, had survived. There was no simple answer.

Twenty-eight days after the operation, Fred was discharged from hospital. He and Carol stayed in the London area for a 90-day period of observation and rehabilitation, and then went home.

Later, back at home, Fred Casswell became honorary chairman of the Saskatchewan Heart Fund and is now a staff member of Transplant International. Today he speaks to many groups as a living example of the miracle of transplants.

WHO IS A POTENTIAL RECIPIENT?

All who have a failed organ are potential transplant recipients, as long as they do not have cancer or a serious infection.

A recipient's age is not a major factor in eligibility. It was once thought that patients under 45 had a better chance of survival. Today, the more important factor is the overall condition of the body. Can the patient's body undergo a major operation, and are the other organs of the body healthy enough to keep functioning after the transplant?

Theoretically in North America, there is no reason why a person who has a nonfunctioning organ should not be able to get on the list of those in need of a transplant. The key is your doctor, who should have all the information regarding diagnosis and referral. Then, if you are assessed as needing a transplant, the transplant center would place your name on the list of potential recipients.

In some instances people are not eligible for a particular kind of transplant. For example, a patient whose heart is diseased but whose lung is also diseased would not receive a heart transplant alone, but rather a heart-lung transplant, because if a lung is defective, a new heart provides no long-term benefit.

Some transplant units have been reluctant to search out a new liver for a patient whose own liver has become diseased through alcoholism. They argue, "Why should we waste a liver — a scarce resource — upon someone whose lifestyle habits could destroy the new organ?" In my opinion, if alcoholics show reasonable evidence of taking steps to deal with their addiction, they should be considered candidates for transplant.

WHO IS A POTENTIAL DONOR?

Most people assume that a donor is probably a young person who has died in an intensive care unit. Such a person is indeed the ideal donor. But in fact the range of donors is much broader.

Everyone is a potential donor of an organ. Consider the donation of eyes. Even a dying individual in advanced old age who wears glasses is a potential donor. For an eye transplant, the age of the donor is irrelevant because, although the entire orbit of the eye is removed, what is actually transplanted is the cornea, the little "window" of the eye through which one sees. The cornea is removed at the morgue or funeral home, put in a preservation fluid and sent to an eye bank. In North America, more than 2 million potential eye donors die each year. If only 10 percent of these became actual donors, we could more than meet the demand for corneal transplants.

For other types of transplants, the donor's age can sometimes make a difference, but even so, not all transplanted organs come from the young. At our hospital, we recently removed the clean, healthy kidneys of a 70-year-old man whose family had given their consent, and gave them to younger patients who were thus freed from dialysis. Generally, however, we prefer kidney donors to be under the age of 60 or 65, and liver and pancreas donors to be under 60. For bone donors, the age range is 16 to 70; for skin donors, 14 to 75; and for heart valves, three months to 55 years.

For a heart transplant, the age of the donor is relatively more specific, because the heart's functioning is so dependent upon the condition of the blood vessels within the heart, and these deteriorate with age. Yet, even this age limit has been expanding so that now we accept donors in their fifties.

The retrieval of several organs and types of tissue from a single donor has become more common, especially when there is enough time to prepare for a multi-organ transplant.

FROM A DONOR FAMILY'S POINT OF VIEW

One day, the morning paper carried the story of a group of teenage boys who had met disaster just outside a small rural community in Ontario. The boys had driven a car down a country road the previous evening. Running in a ditch parallel to the car was a runaway horse. Without warning, the horse jumped from the ditch and landed on the hood of the car. The horrific result: a perfectly healthy 18-year-old had his neck broken and was rushed to intensive care at our hospital, suffering from brain injury, which led, eventually, to brain death.

Later that day I asked the ICU nurse to call me if the neurosurgeon declared the teenager brain-dead. I wanted to approach the boy's family to discuss possible organ donation.

In another part of the hospital lay Clarissa (not real name), only 36 years old, but in desperate need of a new liver. She had been hospitalized, off and on, for several years. Her skin was yellowed from jaundice caused by liver failure, her abdomen was swollen and distended, the rest of her body was emaciated and her gums were starting to bleed. Clarissa's body was being poisoned because her liver was no longer working to cleanse her blood. We feared possible sudden catastrophic bleeding from the esophagus, which patients with cirrhosis of the liver sometimes experience. Sudden bleeding of this nature is one of the most dreaded medical emergencies. Survival for a woman as sick as Clarissa is usually impossible. Her only hope was a liver transplant.

At 3:00 PM a call came from the intensive care unit. The young resident neurosurgeon said, "Dr. Stiller, the young man is brain-dead. I've talked to the family and the father has made it very clear that he doesn't want to donate any of his boy's organs."

"Are you sure?" I asked.

"Yes, I'm sure," the resident responded.

"I'm not so sure," I said. "Experience has shown me it's rare for relatives to refuse when they're approached with gentleness and respect. I'm sure a farmer with a young family will not so quickly say no. In my experience, those who work the land often see the reality of life with greater sensitivity than those boxed in the city. When people are given all the facts, they usually want to participate."

"Well, I've talked to them and they don't want to donate," replied the neurosurgeon.

I paused, then asked, "Would you object if I talked to the family again?"

"No," he said thoughtfully. "I just don't want you crowding them."

"You can be assured I won't do that," I promised.

I accompanied him to the quiet room of the intensive care unit, where the father and mother were sobbing. I spoke gently to the father, asking him when he had last seen his son alive.

The father was guarded and somewhat hostile. After a few moments, he answered my question. As his son had left with his classmates, they had said goodbye, the father offering some last-minute advice about careful driving. Looking forward to a day in London with his classmates, his son had driven off.

I then broached the difficult topic of donation. "Sir, I understand that the neurosurgeon has talked to you about donating your son's organs for transplantation and that you've decided not to. I'm not here to dispute your decision. Rather, I simply want to make sure that you've made that decision based on all the facts."

The father stiffened. "Dr. Stiller, nobody is going to harvest my boy."

I was shocked. Everyone associated with our transplant team was discouraged from using the word "harvest." I am sensitive to how some people are repelled by the idea of organ transplants. For many years, transplantation was considered Orwellian, too bizarre for sound medical practice. Too often, I had heard people refer to me as the "Grim Reaper" of the University Hospital. I deeply resented this label. Instead, I saw myself as a purveyor of life.

I asked, "Where did you hear that?"

"I heard it in the hallway, when they were coming to talk to me. Dr. Stiller, I'm a farmer and I know what harvest means. When we harvest corn, we tear the cob from the stalk. We don't care what happens to the stalk — it just gets trampled under the tires and then thrown away. Nobody is going to harvest my boy."

"Of course not," I assured him. "I'm most disturbed that the term was even used, because we don't harvest here. I grew up in a rural community, too. I know what it is like to work on a farm. And harvesting is not what we do in this hospital. We retrieve life." I decided to try to explain the reality of what goes on in our unit.

"When you came in to see your boy today, I know you were shocked to see his head bandaged and his body still and unconscious. But what gave you hope, as you stood by his bed, was that when you touched him, his skin was still warm. You placed your hand on his wrist and felt his pulse. You looked at the cardiac monitor, saw the tracing, and heard the beep. You also heard the swish of the respirator and saw his chest rise and fall. All of this convinced you that life was still there.

"As a doctor, I too have taken solace in those signs of life.

"You have tended your son throughout the day and were comforted by holding his hand, touching his skin and stroking his forehead. But he hasn't responded. There has been no fluttering of the eyes and no squeezing of the hand. And then you realize that there are no signs that your son even knows you are standing by his bedside. Nevertheless, you tell yourself, there has to be life.

"However, a brain tracing has confirmed the fact that your son's brain is not injured or asleep, not bruised or damaged, but irrevocably dead.

"Your hearts cry out that this can't be so. Your boy is exactly the same as when you first saw him here at the hospital. His skin is warm. His pulse is beating. His chest is rising and falling.

"But your reason affirms that it is just as the specialist has told you. Your son is dead and will never recover. Indeed, the only cause for any evidence of life is the respirator to which he is attached. Reluctantly, you have accepted the facts. You know it is time to turn the respirator off. You want to take your son to the funeral home and from there to his final resting place.

"But even now, the signs of life remain, because there is an enormous amount of life remaining in your son's body. We used to define death as the cessation of heartbeat. Now we know that organs die at different rates. And the brain dies long before many of the other vital organs do. So, as long as the heart is maintained, life in the organs after a fatal injury is exactly the same as it was before. In fact, with the aid of a respirator the heart could function for some time."

But then they asked, "Dr. Stiller, are these real patients who will get these organs, or is it all just for research?"

So I told the grief-stricken parents the other side of the story. "Upstairs on the sixth floor of this hospital is a woman, twice your son's age. She is dying a slow but sure death because her liver has failed. When she dies, there will be no retrievable life in her because, in contrast to what is happening with your son, the death of her liver has made all the rest of her body very sick.

"The same problem applies to a young man living in this city. His heart is slowly ebbing away. He wears a pocket pager, waiting for a call saying that a new heart is available. If he dies, all the life in his body will be gone because his heart, the organ necessary to provide blood to sustain life, will also have died."

I paused to focus my thoughts, and then continued. "I said earlier that we retrieve life in this hospital. Let me tell you what this means. When the decision to transplant is made, the donor and the recipient are taken to the operating room. The donor's body is treated with profound respect, because we are watching one of the most extraordinary acts that a human being can accomplish. The surgical theatre is hushed and reverence for life prevails as the donor organ is removed and taken carefully to the sick, partially destroyed body of the recipient. The sick organ is removed to make way for the new, healthy organ. We watch in silence as the retrieval of life from the donor occurs and the restoration of life in the recipient begins. We watch as the skin begins to clear, the body chemistry begins to improve and the brain gradually quickens as the new organ functions and restores life.

"I'm not asking you to participate in something you think of as harvesting. Rather, I would like you to be a key participant in this wonderful retrieval of life."

I felt the atmosphere in the room change. The meaningless destruction of a healthy teenager — his organs healthy but his brain dead — could be transformed into something meaningful after all.

The father grasped his wife's hand. "Dr. Stiller, can you promise me that's what will happen?"

"Yes, but first I want you to go back and see your son again. Take some time to be sure this is what both of you want to do."

The parents returned to their son's bedside. They touched his hand, still warm. They placed their hands on his chest, still rising and falling with the artificial respiration. They both felt his pulse. But there was no sign of life in the eyes.

When the parents returned to the quiet room, the father spoke: "Dr. Stiller, would you talk to his classmates? They're waiting downstairs." I knew then that he had changed his mind.

The boy's friends had gathered in the waiting room and I explained the transplantation process for them. Many of them wept, but I was deeply moved by their attitude of acceptance. Then the boy's family and friends left the hospital to mourn their loss.

The next day the boy's parish priest called me. "May I tell those who will be attending the funeral what has happened?" he asked.

"Yes," I said. "Tell them a 36-year-old woman facing death is going to live because of a new liver. A 41-year-old man can look forward to a future because of a new heart. Two patients who were tied to an artificial kidney are being released from their prison. Two people who could not see the sun rise in the morning will receive sight. A child suffering from third-degree burns is receiving new skin. And a young man whose knee must be removed will have a joint transplant and will walk again. All because these parents were determined that the death of their son did not have to end only in tragedy."

The priest said he would explain and thanked me.

Several weeks later, the boy's father wrote: "I've lost my son but I take comfort in the knowledge that somewhere out there a part of his life goes on."

The life of this young man will never be replaced. But at least his family knows that out of their pain will come survival for others, because they chose to give the gift of life.

THROUGH THE MEDICAL MAZE

LATE ONE DAY, I received a call from a woman anguished by her life on dialysis. Because of a diseased kidney, she was forced to visit a hospital three times a week, where she was hooked up to a machine to cleanse her blood. This ordeal compromised her job and her household responsibilities. It circumscribed her life and made it impossible for her to travel. She had been waiting for a kidney transplant for three years.

The woman told me that during the past three years, she had been on the hospital's transplant list and that every week when she went for dialysis, she asked her urologist whether an organ might be available. But every week she heard the same old story: no match had been found.

I promised the woman I would check the list of those waiting for a kidney, and then call her back. However, I couldn't find her name. After searching through the potential recipient list for the past three years, I discovered *she had never been registered on the list!* This woman had been waiting in vain for a transplant that would never happen, because her doctor had never ensured that her name was added to the list.

There was no way to explain to the woman what had happened, except to say that her doctor had failed. All of our medical and scientific expertise meant nothing, because her doctor had not entered her name on the waiting list.

The next day the woman called her doctor, who was, of course, embarrassed by his failure to register her. She was tested and judged to be a suitable candidate for a transplant and her name was entered onto the list. *Within four months* she received a new kidney, which is functioning normally today.

THE PATIENT'S RESPONSIBILITY

Recent advances made in the world of medical science are truly phenomenal; nevertheless, patients must keep their eyes open to spot roadblocks within the medical system. All patients have a responsibility to themselves and to their families to find out as much as they can about their disease and its treatment.

For convenience, let me address you, the reader, as if you were a patient needing a transplant. Ask your doctor any unresolved questions. And keep in mind that simply because most medical caregivers seem extremely competent and use long, complicated words, they are not infallible. Doctors may not always appreciate your questions, but you are entitled to ask them.

In order to increase the likelihood of getting a transplant, you must ascertain whether your name is indeed on the transplant list, where it is on the list, and what is being done to find you an organ. Ask your local doctor for the phone number of the transplant center that has the recipients' list on computer file. A phone call will tell you if your name has been entered, the level of urgency assigned to your case, and, often, the number of times there has been a tissue match.

The decision to give an organ to one patient as opposed to another is at times quite subjective. It is important to know who makes the decisions and on what basis decisions are made. Given that we are in the early stages of developing formulas for organ distribution, I advise the patient to actively monitor the system and to ensure for themselves an equal opportunity to receive an organ.

UNDERSTANDING THE TRANSPLANT LIST

How do you get on the organ transplant list? You must first be diagnosed by your doctor as in need of a transplant. When your doctor decides it's time to discontinue treating the diseased organ in favor of procuring a new one, you will be referred to a transplant center. At the center patients are told the facts about transplants, checked to verify that they don't have cancer or infection, and examined to rule out that there is no alternative therapy for the diseased organ. While diagnosis does vary from one doctor to another, increasingly standardized measurements are being used by transplant centers to ensure that all patients are given the same opportunity.

The next important step is to get your name on the transplant list. The doctor at the transplant unit is responsible for ensuring that the person's name, blood group and tissue type are entered into the file, along with the date of entry. The tissue type was determined from a blood sample previously analyzed at the lab.

Each time a donor kidney becomes available, the tissue type of the donor is determined by testing the donor's white blood cells from the spleen, lymph nodes or blood. The serum of all potential kidney recipients is crossmatched against the donor's white cells. Negative crossmatches indicate that the recipient has not formed any antibodies that could reject the kidney. If there's more than one recipient with a negative crossmatch, the recipient whose tissue type most closely resembles the donor's will receive the donor kidney. (Chapter 2 discusses the immune system and rejection of organs.)

It is important to learn the rules governing the transplant list, and to find out how many patients are on the list and, of course, to confirm that you are in fact listed. How can you ensure that you don't encounter the same misfortune as the woman who had been waiting needlessly for three years? Call the transplant center or, better yet, visit it personally. Staff at the center will give you reading material and explain to you how the system works;

they will also doublecheck that you are on the waiting list. Ask how many donor organs are being obtained and the number of transplants being done. This will let you know your status relative to others on the list, and how likely it is that you will receive a transplant within the next few months. Find out whom to contact if you have any questions.

It is important to understand that you are part of an *organ-sharing* program. This program attempts to distribute available organs equitably to those whose tissue matches best, and who therefore have a better chance of success. Unfortunately, this system may mean a longer wait for some people.

Waiting time also depends on the type of organ needed. A heart, heart-lung, or liver transplant is a matter of life and death, so the waiting time is kept to a minimum.

For those in need of a kidney, the situation is less desperate since some patients have survived on dialysis for up to 20 years. Therefore, longer waiting periods for kidney transplants are common, especially since there are more potential recipients waiting. Thus, it is especially vital that someone waiting for a kidney knows the various factors and criteria that go into the process of deciding who gets a donor organ.

It is unfortunately true that in most programs, a patient waiting for a transplant is completely unaware of when a donor organ is potentially available. In the case of a kidney recipient, for example, a number of suitable cross-matches against donor kidneys could be made, but the kidneys could still be given to other patients, with no explanation provided for the choice. However, patients waiting for an organ should be able to find out how often their tissue is tested against potential donors.

THE NATIONAL TRANSPLANT PROGRAM

There are two types of transplant waiting lists. The first comprises many kidney patients who are on dialysis. In some transplant centers, most kidneys that become available are used in that particular center or region; they are seldom sent to transplant centers outside the region unless the donor belongs to an uncommon blood group. The second list, a shorter one, comprises patients waiting for other organs, including liver, heart, lungs and pancreas.

A new rating system instituted in North America indicates the level of urgency for vital organs such as liver, heart and lungs. In Canada the rating system for the liver is "1" to "4" with "4" as the most urgent; for hearts, it is "1" to "6" with "6" as the most urgent. The UNOS rating system is the same for livers; for heart-lung and lung they use an "active" or "inactive" status; for heart they use only "1" and "2," with "1" as the more urgent. Usually patients waiting for a kidney are only rated as "active" or "inactive" (temporarily on hold).

Each list is organized into two categories. The first is the regional category. For example, in Toronto there are four transplant centers for that region. When an organ comes available in one of the centers, it is offered first to those transplant centers within the region. If there is no patient listed as "6" in that region, but a category "6" is located in another region, the organ is offered to the latter. If no category "6" patient is listed, the first region assigns the organ to a category "5" patient. In other words, a local donor tends to be matched with a local recipient first. But livers and lungs are often distributed to the most urgent patient with the longest waiting time, regardless of region.

The supply-demand ratio in a region determines whether patients will get an organ sooner, or later. It is not just the size of the recipient waiting list that determines how soon a transplant can be done. How active the organ donor program is in a particular region is also a factor. If you are on a list in a center that isn't aggressive and successful in receiving donor organs, your chances of getting a transplant in time are reduced, because patients are dependent on the surplus of organs from those regions that are more successful in recruiting organ donations.

Now the second category comes into play. In Canada, the pool of donor organs is managed by an informal network of transplant centers, and in the United States, by the United Network for

Organ Sharing (UNOS). These two systems keep updates on all the potential recipients in all regions.

When patients understand the rating system and know which category they are in, they can find out how many patients in their center are ahead of them and the approximate waiting time for patients in their category. This information is only valid on the day given, however, because the rating of a new patient who has been added to the list may be of greater urgency, thereby shifting the order of the list. Also, if a patient's illness worsens, that person's rating acquires a higher degree of urgency. A patient may be moved from a nonactive, to an active, to an urgent listing, depending upon the seriousness of the case.

The criteria determining whether a patient should be on the active list is based on an assessment by the physician or surgeon in charge of a particular transplant program. Don't assume that because you are told you are next on the list, you will therefore receive the next organ that becomes available. Months later, after other transplants have been done in that center, you might still be waiting for a donor. You can make a rough calculation of your waiting time by examining the number of patients on the list, the various categories assigned, and the number of transplants being done that involve the organ you need. This can help you estimate the likelihood of receiving a transplant in the next six months to a year.

The highest risk period for a patient is before a transplant is performed, not six months afterwards. Thus, while you are waiting, it is essential to know what your priority rating is. If you encounter a long waiting list in a region where the supply of donors clearly does not meet the demand, then it could be to your advantage to register at a center where the list suggests a greater likelihood of an available organ. You can ask your doctor to investigate other regions to determine the number of patients waiting for organs compared with the number of transplants being done at that center or region.

Sometimes the patient may request a transplant, regardless of tissue match. Tired of a prolonged wait, some of my patients have demanded to receive the next available kidney, whether or not the tissue match is exact.

While I advise patients to keep in touch with the transplant unit and to ask every conceivable question, being aggressive will not guarantee receiving a transplant. In fact, the transplant team sometimes perceives overassertiveness as interference.

Sometimes patients feign illness or, conversely, avoid telling the transplant team of their medical problems, fearing an adverse effect on their chances of receiving an organ. These maneuvers are not only counterproductive, but they may also impede a patient's chances of a successful transplant.

THE TRANSPLANT CENTER AND THE TRANSPLANT TEAM

Because organ transplants are done in hospitals, it is vital that recipients understand how hospital systems function.

Hospitals are run by boards of directors, managers, doctors, nurses, technicians and other support staff.

Not long ago, open-heart surgery was the standard by which a health center was judged to be in the forefront of medicine. Today, the symbol of prestige is whether or not a hospital has a transplant unit. Given today's high-tech medicine, it has become fashionable for hospitals to have their own transplant centers. Both university hospitals and large city hospitals are establishing transplant centers to serve the increasing demand for organ transplants.

A hospital's push to open an organ transplant unit has both a positive and a negative aspect. On the one hand, it can encourage the administration, the staff and public supporters to work hard to upgrade the care provided at the hospital. The drive to upgrade also helps generate sensitivity to the need to enter the modern era of extending life by transplantation.

The negative side to the drive to open a transplant unit is the pressure to succeed exerted on the center, especially in the early phases. Obviously, the center wants to demonstrate its legitimacy to the hospital board, the government, the community and charitable institutions, so that funding will continue.

This pressure to succeed could lead a new transplant center to establish a policy of accepting only those transplant cases for whom a positive outcome is most likely. Thus, one patient at a higher risk of not surviving a transplant could be denied one, while another patient whose success is more assured would be accepted.

The opening of a complex, high-profile, multi-organ transplant service in a hospital can have an incredible impact on staff. Initially, the effect on morale is positive. Most staff members have a strong desire to be associated with the multi-organ transplant service. They are enthusiastic, eager and proud to be working with a highly trained and highly motivated team of experts providing a special service to patients whose lives are threatened. But the emotional impact and the stress cannot be underestimated. A transplant unit operates amidst constant emergencies. The stress is disruptive to family and personal life. Aggravating the stress of patient preparation, surgery and aftercare are the emotional ups and downs that nurses and doctors experience along with recipients and their families. Medical staff must work intensively with the donor families, before, during and after transplantation, offering explanation, encouragement and solace.

Establishing a transplant center requires more, therefore, than just the introduction of new surgical procedures. Transplantation is a multi-disciplinary endeavor requiring multi-faceted expertise. A key component in the success of a transplant unit is a highly skilled surgical transplant team.

Transplant specialists are still uncommon throughout the world. Members of a competent transplant team must be experienced in infectious and metabolic diseases, immunology, hematology and psychiatry.

A transplant recipient in a hospital that is just beginning a new transplant program is at increased risk of surgical complications compared with a recipient in an established transplant center. It takes time for a program to deal with its growing pains and to reach its full capabilities. Until that happens, the patient is caught in a learning curve. If this is true of the transplant period, it's even more true of the postoperative period. During this phase, the administration of drugs to suppress rejection and combat infection is extremely critical. At the same time, the patient's wound must heal.

When we began our transplant program in the University Hospital in London, Ontario, we learned through trial and error. Today, I wish I could have the opportunity of treating those early patients again. They were just as much pioneers as we were. Sometimes honest mistakes were made in diagnosing problems or determining the amount or type of drug needed to overcome rejection. But there is no other way for a transplant unit to begin except by struggling.

While you might try to seek out an established transplant center, you may have little choice, especially if you live in an area that happens to have a brand-new center. To go to a center outside your area can be costly and inconvenient.

Seasoned transplant centers have their problems, too. Recently, they have experienced a rapid growth in the sheer volume of transplants. Sometimes they outstrip their capabilities and resources, which had originally been designed to handle a much smaller program.

It is important for both patient and family to assess the competence and experience of a center before placing the patient's life in the hands of the transplant team. Theoretically, it is possible to choose the hospital in which the operation will take place. Ask the staff at the transplant center to show you the statistics outlining success and failure at that center. Your doctor will recommend a specialist to walk you through the center's screening process. If, after your name is on the list, you select a different hospital, you will have to undergo the time-consuming screening process again.

Choosing a surgeon, other than the one supplied by the transplant center, is also difficult. Unless you strongly prefer to have another surgeon, it is best to stay with the surgeon assigned by the transplant unit.

ORGAN DISTRIBUTION

What is involved in deciding who receives an organ? The decision is based on a number of factors, including blood group, tissue type, the recipient's proximity to the transplant center, how long a patient has been waiting, and most important of all, the clinical assessment of the patient's urgency rating and which recipients promise the best results. Choosing a recipient is a tremendously difficult responsibility resting on the physician or surgeon in charge of the case.

A mental image of the patient and the most recent encounter with that person are clear in the physician's mind when deciding who should receive an available organ. Some patients are more attractive, in a clinical sense, than others, if they have a greater potential for success. While one life cannot be weighed against another, one person's medical needs may simply be more urgent.

Over the years the criteria for determining who should get a transplant have changed. When a brand-new transplant procedure is introduced, only the sickest patients are accepted. This is based on the principle that if death is inevitable and imminent, an attempt at saving that life using a new, unproven procedure is legitimate. As the transplant procedure proves successful, it is offered to patients who are less ill. The criteria for accepting patients shift from the sickest ones to those whose illness may not be as advanced.

Limited to only a few patients because of the lack of donor organs, transplants were once commonly distributed on the basis of "nonmedical" criteria. When dialysis was first introduced, young, professional white males tended to be selected first. Committees comprising both medical staff and lay persons judged which individual was most worthy of this limited resource.

In 1968, Dr. John Dossetor, a pioneer in organ transplantation in Canada, analyzed ten years' worth of data concerning kidney transplants in Montreal. Records showed that although male recipients significantly outnumbered female recipients, the transplant survival rate was higher among women. One explanation for their higher survival rate was that women received more blood transfusions than men. This presumably conditioned their immune systems to accept a foreign tissue. Ironically, women required more blood transfusions because they were kept waiting on dialysis for a transplant longer than men were.

This bias towards males may not have been intentional, but nonetheless, because men were considered the breadwinners in families, they were pushed ahead on the list. And since dialysis units were scarce, first priority was given to those patients most likely to show measurable benefit to society by returning to work and paying taxes.

Dr. Carl Kjellstrand, a noted kidney specialist from Stockholm who once lived in Minneapolis, studied transplantation in the United States, Sweden and Canada. He wrote, "Rich before Poor, Men before Women, White before Black and Young before Old," and claimed that there is a 60 percent greater likelihood of receiving a kidney transplant for patients in one of these four "favored" groups.

Some health economists argue that it makes better sense financially to give a heart or kidney to a 30-year-old rather than a 60-year-old, even though in Canada the Charter of Rights and Freedoms prohibits discrimination on the basis of age. In my experience, physical disabilities and diseases such as diabetes can affect decisions concerning who receives an organ. Shocking as it may seem, the disabled may be considered too dependent on society and a diabetic may be seen as being too compromised health-wise for long-term success.

Unless a patient chooses not to accept a transplant because of other disabling diseases, then factors such as sex, age, race and ability to pay — especially in countries like Canada that have an equitable medical plan — should have nothing to do with select-

ing organ recipients. Transplant centers must clearly demonstrate unbiased criteria for accepting people into transplant
programs and distributing organs.

As noted earlier, medical personnel sometimes regard a person who incurs illness through abuse as a less worthy recipient.
For example, an alcoholic in need of a liver transplant might be
perceived as likely to return to alcohol, thus not only destroying
another liver but also hurting the reputation of transplants.
However, statistics show that less than 20 percent of liver recipients who were alcoholic prior to the transplant revert to alcoholism. If self-inflicted disease were a criterion prohibiting certain
people from having transplants, then those who are overweight,
sedentary, smoke and have heart disease would be denied a new
organ. Except for objective factors such as tissue type, blood type
and organ size, nothing should jeopardize equal rights for organ
recipients.

The medical community must identify all relevant factors and
criteria and document them in such a way that if called on to
defend their judgment before peers or a court of law, the
rationale for selecting a recipient can be clearly discerned.
However, in moments of doubt, the decision to confer an organ
to one patient as opposed to another is usually based on which
patient has waited longer or needs it the most.

Theoretically, any patient waiting for a liver and in category
"4" — on life-support systems in an ICU and facing death unless
a new organ is obtained — should be next in line each time.
What actually happens is that the location of the patient and the
location of the available organ greatly influence the decision.
Whether a locally retrieved organ is used locally for a very urgent
patient, or given to an organ pool and therefore distributed to
the most urgent case on that list, is often determined by the
director of the transplant program, who must keep the distribution criteria in mind.

Some patients are on a transplant list in a center or a region
where an adequate donor program is not in place and the
likelihood of receiving a transplant is reduced. In Canada, the

network of transplant centers, and in the U.S., the United Network for Organ Sharing (UNOS) attempt to combat this problem. Before these systems existed, there was no means whereby the most urgent patients would receive an organ if there was no organ available in the immediate region.

Different rules govern the distribution of different organs, for example, liver, kidney and heart. And an added unknown is how the local center applies those rules.

One major problem is: Who owns the organ once it has been removed from the donor's body? Some think the organ is held in trust by the surgeon or physician in charge of the retrieval program. The doctor entrusted with the organ is responsible for choosing a recipient. However, a complication arises in defining whether the physician's responsibility in making a choice is limited to the local hospital, program, region, country or the world. As technology enhances the capacity to transport organs over greater distances and to sustain them longer, the perspective on this problem will become increasingly global.

If the transplant scene resembles a maze to you, don't be intimidated. Whether you are a person in need of a transplant or a relative or close friend of a potential recipient, be assertive in learning all you can about the process. Remember that organ transplants are the goal of medical specialists who are deeply committed to meeting the physical and emotional needs of a patient languishing in need of a transplant. Keep as up-to-date as possible with technological advances in transplant science, as well as with the particulars of your own situation. Your life may depend upon not getting lost in a bureaucratic maze.

THE DOCTOR AS ROADBLOCK

I**N TODAY'S HEALTH CARE SYSTEM,** patients are reliant on physicians for their physical and often mental well-being. Transplantation is no exception. Whether advising an ailing patient about the option of transplant therapy, or discussing organ donation with a bereaved family, the physician is in a pivotal position. Without information and support from the attending physician, a transplant is unlikely to take place.

Whereas a well-informed doctor can be an asset, a skeptical doctor can be a roadblock to transplantation. Too often a transplant is stonewalled by doctors who don't give their patients sufficient information. Far too many patients die without knowing about the option of an organ transplant.

Too often, a physician's view is that transplantation is an experimental procedure, carried out in a few select hospitals where patients live only a few weeks or months, and where little long-term benefit for patients is derived. Nothing could be further from the truth. Every day, waiting rooms are filled with patients who have had transplants — heart, liver, kidney, cornea and bone — and who are leading healthy, productive lives. Recipients include fathers, mothers, babies, physicians, nurses, lawyers, teachers, artists, truck drivers and business people.

They write me from ski slopes and from scuba diving trips,

brimming with gratitude for their restored vitality and the prospect of a normal and healthy tomorrow. Invariably, during their yearly checkups, they express their deep gratitude for the unknown donor who has renewed their lives.

A SECOND CHANCE

Patients with heart failure are completely dependent upon their physician's advice as to the best course of therapy. If, in the mind of the attending physician, transplantation is neither worthwhile nor accessible, the prognosis will be, "Nothing more can be done." In such cases patients are not adequately informed and are therefore unable to make an educated decision about their own well-being.

Here is a story concerning a 23-year-old university student from the Maritimes who almost died because his doctor did not inform him of the available options.

Late one summer, Ken decided to travel west for the first time to visit friends. An avid athlete, Ken enjoyed the outdoors and spent much of his time hiking, bicycling and playing squash. His friends knew him as someone who loved life.

One morning during his holiday he felt some discomfort. He assumed that a flu he had had recently was lingering on. But the family with whom he was staying were concerned about his noticeable shortness of breath. Finally, Ken went to the emergency department at the hospital in the city he was visiting. The emergency physician was alarmed. Ken's chest x-ray showed a heart more than twice its normal size.

Dismayed, Ken realized that this flu-like illness represented the onset of a serious heart ailment. Medical terms such as "myocarditis" and "cardiomyopathy" meant little to him, but he knew they spelled trouble. Underlying his disappointment over an interrupted vacation was a nagging fear that here was something he was not about to get out of easily.

One night about two months later, as he wrestled feelings of despair and frustration, Ken overheard a conversation in the hospital corridor. The word "transplant" was mentioned, but Ken assumed that someone else was being discussed. Fortunately for Ken, *he* was the subject of discussion. Until then, Ken and his family had been told that although some patients recovered from this type of heart disease, the majority did not, and that for Ken, survival was unlikely.

The internist in charge of Ken's case had gone on holiday. Why hadn't he suggested a transplant? Perhaps he had participated in an unsuccessful transplant and had therefore concluded that such a procedure was out of the question. Or he may have undergone medical training during the post-Barnard era, when many medical scientists became cynical about transplants.

When the nurse in charge conferred with the on-call chief of staff, she mentioned the word "transplant." The chief of staff threw up the usual roadblocks: "What are his chances anyway? The only place he could get a transplant would be at some far-off hospital. The list is too long and he would only die waiting. Can this family afford the terrible expense involved? The procedure is so experimental, we are probably doing the patient a favor by not mentioning it."

The nurse protested this attitude. She had been trained at London's University Hospital, where she had seen young dying patients restored to normal life by the replacement of a diseased heart. But she recognized that no one at this western hospital had been directly involved in a successful transplant. Luckily, however, she knew that a young and aggressive cardiologist in town had been trained in the same hospital where she had worked. Perhaps he could give a more positive prognosis.

Despite the chief physician's misgivings, Ken was transferred to the care of the young cardiologist, whose pronouncement was swift: Ken's only hope for survival was to receive a new heart.

A new heart: the sound of these words both frightened and exhilarated Ken. When we were told the facts of Ken's condition over the phone, we agreed he should be brought to University Hospital in London immediately.

When we saw Ken, it was obvious he had only a short time to

live. Although other patients were on the list before him, Ken urgently needed immediate attention.

Ken arrived on Wednesday. He received a heart transplant on Sunday. Within a week he stood outside his room in the intensive care unit. We were delighted with the tremendous change in his color, breathing and mental functioning. But a mere three-day delay in the decision to bring him to London would have completely sabotaged his chances.

Seventeen months after his heart transplant, Ken stood at the head table of the Great Hall at the University of Western Ontario, resplendent in a rented tuxedo. He shared the dais with the Honorable Jake Epp, then Canada's Minister of Health and Welfare. This young heart recipient had been chosen to pay tribute to Professor Jean Francois Borel, discoverer of the anti-rejection drug, cyclosporine.

It seemed so very appropriate that Ken should rub shoulders with the man whose discovery had promised him a long and full life. Ken — who like most transplant recipients is dependent on the drug for survival — concluded his remarks with, "Thank you, Dr. Borel, with all my heart."

MISCONCEPTIONS AND SKEPTICISM AMONG DOCTORS

The obstacles that Ken had to overcome were erected largely by the medical profession and the hospital system. Financial, geographic, legal or ethical barriers did not play a role in depriving Ken of an immediate transplant referral. Rather, the barrier was the perception of Ken's physician and the consulting cardiologist that transplantation was not in Ken's best interests.

There are some basic reasons why some doctors are slow to recommend a transplant for a patient. The major reason is that they think organ transplants are still an unproven treatment. Although thousands of transplants are being done each year in North America, many family doctors are trapped by a conservative mentality that can hinder any profession: "If we haven't done it this way before, it must not be worthwhile." The medical community's basic orientation has been to retard or reverse disease by medication, or to remove disease by surgery. It is difficult to change this mindset.

The second reason for doctors' reluctance to recommend a transplant is that many of today's doctors graduated from medical school before organ transplants were taught. The rapid advances of scientific technology have caught not only the average citizen by surprise, but have also surprised those within the medical profession. Not only does the public sometimes think of organ transplants as a new and experimental space-age medicine; but also physicians who have not had direct contact with successful recipients view transplants with a great deal of skepticism. For a doctor steeped in the old ways of practicing medicine, it is not easy to cross the bridge of modern technology and, in the highly charged moment of encroaching death, to talk about transplant procedures, especially if the doctor believes they are highly risky and experimental.

A significant number of my medical colleagues question the future benefits and availability of transplantation. As a result, even though today most organs are transplanted with a success rate of 70 to 75 percent or better, the majority of patients with failing organs will not receive new ones.

Until recently, professional medical societies did not consider transplantation sufficiently effective to offer training programs related to it. Medical societies (especially the fee-setting societies, such as provincial medical associations in Canada and Medicare in the United States) and, until recently, most insurance companies, did not provide a recognized fee to the medical profession for transplantation procedures.

TRANSPLANTS AS LEGITIMATE TREATMENT

In my 20 years as a physician and scientist, I have never seen another medical procedure under such constant pressure to prove its legitimacy to the medical profession as transplantation has been. Time after time we have had to prove that organ transplants are scientifically sound, ethically legitimate and, as well, that they provide a source of emotional healing to bereaved families. To demand that a certain success rate be achieved before transplantation is considered a legitimate therapy is, in my view, irrational. The brutal fact is, for someone with a diseased heart, the only alternative, apart from receiving a heart transplant, is death.

It is a paradox that doctors who reject organ transplants as a viable therapy often treat patients suffering from fatal diseases for which there is much less real or statistical hope, for when given the opportunity to replace diseased, transplantable organs, we can promise that a minimum 75 percent of recipients will lead restored lives. For example, statistics show that patients with cancer of the esophagus, stomach, colon or kidney have a 5 to 50 percent chance of surviving a maximum of five years.

Because of the widespread incidence of cancer, a high percentage of families have been touched by it. As a result, people are relatively familiar with modern forms of cancer therapy. Thus, when the dread word "cancer" is stated by the family doctor, the family or community supports the individual in the search for treatment. The usual expectation is that in a short time a specialist will be found, the patient will be told the odds of survival, and treatment will be undertaken.

Sometimes a cancer patient elects not to undergo therapy because of the pain of treatment or the low survival odds. But this response is rare. Usually, most people seize on any opportunity for extended life and accept the therapy, even though it may involve pain and discomfort without a sure guarantee of recovery.

Isn't it odd, therefore, that where transplantation is concerned the reverse philosophy is applied? The view seems to be that if you can't guarantee a high level of success (and that success is measured not only in terms of survival but also in terms of a patient's return to work), then hospitals won't provide the service, insurance companies won't pay for it and governments won't give their approval. When a patient is told, for example, that he has hepatitis (viral infection of the liver) and irreparable cirrhosis, the doctor's immediate response should be, "Where can I get that liver replaced?" Instead, because of the skepticism pervading the medical community, some doctors assume that the likelihood of success is so small, the chances of obtaining a donor in time so remote and the cost so unjustified, that it is useless to even suggest an organ transplant to the patient.

It is curious that medical ethicists and health economists extol the virtues of using society's dollars to meet human needs, but nevertheless call for a rationing of money for transplantation, a branch of medicine that actually extends life and reduces medical costs.

If, after informing a patient of a cancer diagnosis, a doctor did not refer the patient to a cancer specialist to have the tumor removed and proper cancer therapy instituted, this omission would constitute malpractice. If, after informing a patient that a hopelessly diseased organ could be replaced, a doctor did not refer the patient to a transplant center for examination and a possible organ transplant, would that not also constitute malpractice? How can we reconcile a modern medical system — in which there is virtually instantaneous communication — with the fact that patients are allowed to die of disorders that are treatable, in facilities that are accessible, when potential donors are available?

THE COSTS

Some politicians and medical staff complain that the cost of doing a transplant is so high that it takes much-needed money away from other forms of medicine.

It is true that developing transplant technology and training personnel necessitates extra funding. Most hospitals are already struggling for funds and establishing an organ transplant unit strains financial resources all the more.

Staffing costs for a new transplant center are heavy and unpredictable. Operating-room nursing staff must be available at all times. Intensive care nurses must be ready to provide concentrated nursing care both immediately after a transplant operation and during the recovery phase. Both before and after the transplant, the services of physiotherapists, social workers, psychologists, blood bank personnel and pharmaceutical staff are needed.

Finally, there is the high cost of retrieving organs. A well-paid retrieval team and expensive jet travel are needed to retrieve an organ as quickly as possible.

However, once a transplant unit is under way, the cost of treating a patient who has a failed organ compared with doing an organ transplant is much higher. While some people suggest that, because of the high cost of transplantation, medical dollars should be allocated to research and prevention instead, facts reveal a different picture. Setting aside the incalculable cost of suffering, let's look at one example. Keeping a kidney patient alive on dialysis costs $28,175 per year. (Amounts discussed are in U.S. dollars.) The cost of a kidney transplant is $37,481.[*] While the annual cost of dialysis goes on indefinitely, following a once-only transplant cost, the annual cost for cyclosporine treatment is only $6,000 to $7,000 per year.[†]

In a study of 50 kidney patients who were taken off dialysis and given a transplant, there were savings of $887,879 within four years.[*]

In Canada, the cost of transplants is completely covered by Provincial medical plans. Cost is not an issue for the recipient or the family of the donor. If your doctor recommends that you should have a transplant, and if the transplant center approves, cost will not enter into the decision when an organ becomes available.

[*]   Optenberg, S.A. and G.J. Jaffers, "A Prospective Cost Comparison Between Renal Transplantation and Chronic Hemodialysis at Wilford Hall Medical Center," *Military Medicine*, 1986; 151 (12): 630-633.
[†]   Moskop, J.C. "The Moral Limits to Federal Funding for Kidney Disease," *Hastings Center Report*, April 1987, pp. 11-15.

THE DOCTOR'S DILEMMA

THE PRESSURES ON DOCTORS today are enormous and the expectations high. Many patients expect their doctor to be a psychologist, minister and friend. All medical staff, especially family doctors, work under a great deal of stress. Yet those of us who specialize in organ transplants urge our colleagues to venture beyond what they were taught in medical schools and to incur an additional stress — namely, to initiate the process of organ procurement.

The viewpoint of one's doctor regarding organ donations is critical in the decision to donate the organs of a loved one. In a survey of families of organ donors entitled "Kind Strangers: The Families of Organ Donors" (reported in *Health Affairs*, Summer 1987, pp. 35-47), researchers Helen Batten and Jeffrey Prottas identified the role of doctors in helping a family to decide on organ donation. Fifty percent of respondents said that their family doctor had influenced their decision to donate the organ of their loved one.

For most families, the moment of decision arrives very soon after the death of their loved one. In the Batten and Prottas study, 57 percent of those who decided to donate an organ made the decision within one hour of a relative's death. Another 24 percent did so within 24 hours.

For everyone involved, the tension in a life-and-death situation is extremely high. The doctor must respond quickly but with acute sensitivity. Unless the hospital has a patient in critical condition waiting for an organ, it is unlikely that a doctor will take time out of a busy schedule to talk about a subject that could upset or offend the patient's family. If the hospital has no written transplantation policy, the need to discuss an organ donation with a family in shock will probably be low on a doctor's list of priorities.

FROM THE PHYSICIAN'S POINT OF VIEW

I was reminded of the personal side of the conflicts confronting a doctor when I received a call from a colleague who practices medicine in Ontario. Before I tell you about the call, let me first provide a background to the conversation . . .

It had been a long day and the waiting room was oppressive with the early September heat. The fragrance of the colognes and perfumes worn by the 14 patients who had entered the examining room that afternoon predominated over the antiseptic smell of the nurses' preparation room.

In his mid-50s, Dr. George Kennedy* was a well-regarded neurologist, well liked by patients and referring physicians. His eyes focused on the patient in the examining room. He gently prompted the patient to describe her symptoms. As he tactfully posed questions and elicited answers, he was able to piece together a complicated neurological analysis.

As he listened to the patient, he glanced briefly out the window and noted wisps of cloud drifting across the sky. He thought fleetingly of his sailboat up at the marina. He hoped to be on her by six o'clock. His wife, Laura, had invited her sister and brother-in-law to stay overnight. He calculated the amount of time it would take to see the next two patients and still give him enough

---

* This is not a true story; rather, it reflects a hypothetical situation.

time to get to the marina before his family arrived.

The phone rang. The secretary responded, "I'm sorry, Dr. Kennedy is with a patient right now. Can he call you back?" There was a pause and then he heard her say, "Sorry, Dr. Sinclair, of course I'll put you through right away." She buzzed the intercom. Dr. Kennedy stepped out of the examining room and picked up the phone.

It was his student resident calling from the hospital. One of Kennedy's patients, only 29 years old, lay in the intensive care unit. She had been admitted 48 hours earlier, after developing an acute headache followed by unconsciousness; there was bleeding from an aneurysm in the brain. Upon arrival at the hospital, she was already unresponsive. The admitting doctor had written on the chart that there seemed to be little chance of recovery.

In the intensive care unit, the respirator and intravenous fluids continued to support the woman's body, but medical staff watched helplessly as her brain deteriorated. Nothing could be done. The bleeding had already destroyed the vital parts of the brain and no surgical correction was possible. The inevitable ending: a declaration of brain death.

Dr. Kennedy was not surprised by the call. But the timing was terrible: with only two more patients to see, he would have just enough time to drive to the cottage.

He calculated how long it would take to drive to the hospital, do what needed to be done, handle the relatives in a kind and thoughtful way, and still arrive home on time.

He told his secretary that the last two patients would have to be rescheduled. He quickly wrapped up his examination and dictated a report to the referring doctor. He rushed to the hospital. Nothing seemed to go right: the lights were against him and the five o'clock traffic was slow. When he arrived at the hospital his parking space was taken, forcing him to find a place in the visitor's parking lot. The intensive care unit was on the second floor. He took two steps at a time, thinking that unless he was in his car in 35 minutes, he would upset the evening's plans.

His patient was precisely as the resident had described. She was on a respirator, the intravenous was dripping and the heart monitor showed a normal cardiographic tracing. The resident informed him that he had examined the patient thoroughly and all clinical tests showed no sign of any brain activity.

Dr. Kennedy noticed that in the isolation room in the intensive care unit was a patient waiting for a liver transplant. He realized that his patient was a potential organ donor.

He thought about the arduous and time-consuming process of explaining to the family not only the circumstances of the death of their sister, wife and daughter, but also all the questions that would tumble out of a discussion of organ donation. What would such a discussion do for this patient and her family? Surely it would make them suffer more and disrupt the process of grieving and disposing of the body. He knew that to initiate the discussion meant at least another hour or two. He studied the patient's chart and noted that all of the criteria for death had been met. After examining the patient, he said to the nurse and the resident, "I think the respirator should be turned off. I'll talk to the family. It is obvious that brain death has occurred."

The nurse looked at him expectantly. "Do you think we should ask about organ donation?" she asked. Dr. Kennedy flipped to a temperature graph in the chart and noted that a fever had been present within the past 24 hours. Without looking at the nurse, he said, "I don't think she is a suitable donor. She has had a fever in the past 24 hours and may be infected. And in any event, I think this family has suffered enough."

Dr. Kennedy turned towards the waiting family . . .

A while later, as he drove from the hospital, Dr. Kennedy knew that he should have done more. The woman's eyes were good. Her heart was young and healthy, and because she was under 30 her lungs could have been used. Her liver was normal and she would have been an ideal kidney donor. On the other hand, he wondered, perhaps that fever really was an impediment . . . In any event, it was over now and he had to be at the cottage in time to meet his family and friends.

The next morning I received the call from George Kennedy. "Cal," he asked, "tell me, how important is fever in eliminating someone as a donor? If a patient has a fever, which means they had infection, wouldn't it eliminate them as a potential donor because of what might be transmitted to the recipient?"

My first thought was, "I wonder if George had a donor or is thinking about someone in the past?" So I said, "Well, do you have a donor, George?"

"No, no," he protested, "I just wanted it for my information."

I explained that fever sometimes reflects infection and if there were evidence of a serious systemic infection in which bacteria were invading all the potential organs, we probably would not accept a donor's organs.

"In any event," I said, "as you know, George, most individuals have fever when their brain is crushed, which is a reflection of tissue damage. We usually ignore that if there isn't good evidence of infection."

There was a pause and I somehow felt that he wished my answer had been different. "Thanks very much, Cal. I'll tell the residents and nurses about that when we're dealing with potential donors."

THE DOCTOR'S DILEMMA: RESPONSIBILITY AFTER DEATH

Dr. Kennedy's reaction was more than a conflict of personal versus professional commitments. It was a reluctance to enter into a new era of medical practice. Just as doctors in the early years of this century had to reformat their thinking about disease and its treatment, so today medical practitioners must learn to think differently and to accept the emotional challenges involved in transplantation.

Anticipating the death of a patient when the vital organs are still healthy is foreign to medical tradition. To approach the family of a dying patient with a request for organ donation requires increased emotional contact with the grieving family, a stress which a doctor may be reluctant to face. Taking the time and energy to explain the rationale for organ donation and how the process works is more than some doctors are prepared to do.

There is also the issue of not wanting to offend the family. The patient and family believe the physician's prime interest is the well-being of the patient and the needs of the family. In the moments following death, the family members are often in a tight circle, holding hands, crying and exchanging words of support and condolence. Having just announced the sad news of death, a doctor is reluctant to say: "I've got another idea. Why not donate an organ from your loved one?" The subject seems too jarring and disrespectful. If the doctor has not had an opportunity to broach the possibility of organ donation earlier, it is not easy to break the tight seal of the grieving family's emotional circle. An abrupt reference to organ donation might lead the family to conclude that the doctor lacks sensitivity and that their interests are no longer his.

In the past, doctors have been taught that their responsibility to the patient ends at death. At that time, they hand the body over to a coroner or funeral director and the relatives turn to a rabbi, priest or minister. Traditionally, there has been no responsibility to consider the wishes of the deceased. Asking a doctor to assume those responsibilities and raising the delicate question of organ donation is too much for some.

In addition, the doctor's emotions, which often go unrecognized by both patients and physicians themselves, do play a role. Physicians may feel a combination of defensiveness and grief over the death of a patient. After all, their responsibility is to deal with a patient's medical problem. They have entered into a contractual relationship with the patient with the aim of restoring health. When this relationship fails, due to either an inevitably fatal injury or the inadequacy of currently available therapy, a doctor may internalize a sense of failure. Sometimes this is accompanied by deep grief, especially if a close involvement with the patient has developed over the course of a long and serious illness. While the physician is extending consolation to the relatives, in a very real sense the physician may also be seeking consolation.

A doctor's discussion with relatives after the death of a patient is usually brief and formal. The focus tends to be on the patient's illness and the inevitability of death and, in some cases, on how tragic it would have been for the patient to have survived in a vegetative state. There may be little discussion of what constitutes a diagnosis of brain death or the process leading up to it. That discussion is difficult for both the relatives and the physician.

A doctor tends not to prolong discussions following the death of a patient. In fact, a doctor wants to move on to other patients where the successes of practicing medicine may be enjoyed. A doctor would much rather leave a dead patient to the coroner, and the relatives to the psychologist, social worker or clergy.

Physicians thrive on successes, not failures. A foray into a discussion of organ donation not only adds to the complexity of the moment but is also time-consuming. It involves explaining the process, getting consent and signing forms. Then the physician must attend to details such as the dead patient's blood pressure, respiration and body chemistry. This occurs when the physician is no longer carrying out the original contract with the patient, that of restoring life. In such a situation, it is difficult for the physician and nurses to maintain their sense of commitment and excitement as they emotionally regroup and view the brain-dead patient in a different light.

THE PHYSICIAN'S POWER OVER LIFE

The key to successful organ donation is for the physician to anticipate the brain death of an individual before it occurs, so the organs can be kept viable with a respirator. Once the heart has stopped, death creeps throughout the rest of the body. It is the doctor's responsibility to ensure that the body of the donor remains on the respirator and that health in the organs is maintained until a medical team can retrieve the organ(s). With the heart, liver and kidneys, death ensues within a matter of minutes. An organ cannot be transplanted from someone whose heart has stopped for 30 minutes. When the cells begin to die, the process is irreversible.

It is tragic when a physician, reluctant to assume the responsibility of asking for donation, makes the decision not to preserve the deceased's body for organ donation without consulting the family.

I will never forget the appalling experience of Judy. She and her family had moved to Canada, where her husband, John, had accepted a new job. One morning, sitting at his desk, John experienced an excruciating pain in his head. He fell to the floor in convulsions. After being rushed to hospital, he was put on a respirator in the intensive care unit and then examined. A burst blood vessel had destroyed the brain matter and brain death was almost certain. Doctors and nurses attempted to reduce the brain swelling by giving cortisone and fluids.

Judy was told there was a likelihood of brain death, although doctors assured her they would carefully observe her husband overnight and would do all they could.

Judy maintained a vigil at her husband's bedside, realizing that the life they had looked forward to was over. She tried to put her husband's imminent death into some sort of perspective.

Sleep did not come to Judy that night. She lay for awhile on the vinyl couch in the waiting room, recalling things that were important to her and her husband. Later, she slipped back into the ICU. She was struck by the fact that her husband looked just as he had only 24 hours ago, when he lay asleep in their bed, his body warm to her touch.

As the hours passed, Judy reflected upon what had motivated this wonderful man. He had never been a man impassioned by causes, although he cared deeply about people. And for some reason he felt very strongly about one issue. On several occasions he had signed a donor card, remarking to Judy that should he die in such a way that his organs and tissues could be used, he wanted them to be donated. Here was an opportunity for John to demonstrate his interest in helping other people in one final meaningful act.

Throughout the night, Judy's sense of purpose deepened. She resolved to see that her husband's wish would be honored.

At seven in the morning, a nurse came up from intensive care and said, "Judy, the doctor is examining your husband and he'll be out shortly to talk to you."

Although she anticipated bad news from the doctor, Judy was strengthened by a sense that all was not lost.

After 90 minutes, the doctor finally arrived and spoke with her.

"I'm so sorry, Judy, but your husband is dead."

She faltered for a moment. Her anticipation of those final words could not prepare her for the impact of the words themselves.

Then she said, "I knew that would be the diagnosis. But one thing I do want is to have his organs used. Maybe his heart could help someone else. Maybe his kidneys could take somebody off an artificial kidney machine. Maybe his liver could be transplanted to someone dying of a diseased liver."

The doctor looked at her anxiously. "I'm sorry, he is not a suitable donor."

Judy couldn't believe what she was hearing.

"I don't understand. Why wouldn't he be a suitable donor?"

The doctor replied, "The respirator was turned off over an hour ago so I don't think his organs will be useable."

Judy rushed to the bed where her husband's body now lay cold. She grasped his hand. A wave of grief swept over her. Grief exceeding that of loss. It was now laced with anger. Her husband had been denied an opportunity to carry out his last wish.

Judy left the hospital filled with rage. She too had been denied. The grieving process was now doubly bitter for her.

An intelligent and caring woman, Judy turned her loss and anger into a positive force. In the months that followed, she publicized her experience on CBC's "The Journal," articulating the rights of the donor and the donor's family: the right to give; the right to participate in the decision to donate organs after death; the right to share the gift of life. Those wishes should be respected just as much as matters of inheritance specified in a patient's will.

Judy's efforts have begun a movement that has affected physicians and, most importantly, hospital boards. Because of her determination, other people will not be disappointed.

WHO ASKS?

January 9, 1986

Dear Dr. Stiller,

I am writing to you after attending a presentation on organ donation. . . . My brother-in-law, Walter, was a little less than a month short of his 19th birthday when he was involved in an accident on his motorcycle. The driver was neither impaired nor in a hurry. It was just an accident! It could have been me in that car and we think of the driver with sympathy often, hoping that she has the same kind of support our family has had.

Walter had a broken wrist, suspected internal injuries and, of course, a head injury. He had landed on his back on the pavement and his helmet came off. . . . By morning he was unconscious, but not comatose. Over the next two days he would be occasionally semiconscious, with no understanding of where he was or why he was there. . . .

The following morning around 11 AM his brain hemorrhaged, causing a seizure, and his heart stopped beating. . . . The next 24 hours were an incredible assault on our emotions. We would certainly never have thought of organ donation on our own. At one point after my husband signed the authorization [consent] papers with Walter's father, I had to explain that they weren't going to give Walter a new heart, but that his heart was to go to another person.

At noon, a day after the seizure, four days after the accident, Walter was declared clinically dead. . . . The family gathered together the following day after a visit to the funeral home. If a stranger had looked in on this scene, he would have thought we were celebrating a miracle. We hugged, we kissed and we cried. We were so proud of Walter. Even in death his quiet unassuming generosity was still alive. On the day of the funeral, a friend of ours on the police force called to let us know that the heart recipient was doing very well and was setting records for recovery. This gave our whole family a lot of faith for getting through that day.

We received a letter from the mother of the pancreas recipient but didn't meet Maureen [the heart recipient] until a little over a year later. . . . My husband and I went to their [Maureen's] home in Winnipeg. We almost fell over when there on the TV was a picture of their teenage son and beside that a picture of our brother, Walter. On Christmas Eve a thank-you letter from Maureen appeared in the local paper. I couldn't have asked for a better Christmas present than to know someone I have loved and lost is still remembered.

Bonnie Langeveld

When a fatal accident occurs, the family's usual response is either disbelief or anger or both. At this highly charged time, in the quiet room of the intensive care unit, a sense of despair envelops everyone when the physician pronounces a verdict of brain death.

This "suspended state" — in which the patient is dead neurologically but still functions physiologically with the aid of a respirator — is one that generates enormous distress for both relatives and staff. The sooner the body is taken to the morgue and the relatives can go home to mourn their loss, the sooner everyone can experience some relief.

However, in the midst of crisis there is always a fleeting opportunity for a decisive member of the medical team to suggest the possibility of organ donation to save the lives of others. A spark of charity ignited by a physician, nurse, social worker or chaplain can help to refocus the attention of the grieving relatives. Organ donation gives the next of kin an opportunity to make the deceased's last act a noble one.

A believing doctor is usually one who has seen the benefits of an organ transplant, either in the course of training or through a patient referral. As doctors face a patient's inevitable death, they must consider how to maintain the life-support systems in such a way that the vital organs will remain in good condition for transplantation. Instead of grieving at the loss of the patient — although this will and should occur — the believing doctor will bear in mind the many benefits that can be passed on to other patients.

EDUCATING THE FACILITATORS

All of this drama turns on the efforts of a single person: the one who thinks of organ donation in time. The door of opportunity is narrow. It opens when the possibility of brain death is suspected. If organ donation is not anticipated during this time, it may soon be too late; once brain death has occurred, care must be taken to ensure that body organs continue to function. (Chapter 11 discusses brain death in more detail.)

Who is the key facilitator in this process? The decision to approach the family usually lies in the hands of the physician, neurologist or neurosurgeon in charge of the case. But any member of the health care team looking after the brain-injured patient may initiate the discussion.

When life for a patient is no longer possible, the physician's response should always be: "Can we help someone else? Is this patient a potential donor?" As part of the normal course of events, attending medical personnel should ask the patient's relatives, "Would you consider donating the organs to save someone else?"

From my life-long work in the medical community, I know that most doctors harbor a deep concern for and commitment towards their patients. A transplant unit must strive to promote each physician's commitment to the process of organ donation as well. And in order to win physicians' support for organ donations, doctors must be educated about transplantation.

Because transplantation is a relatively new branch of medicine, very few physicians have been trained in the transplant process. It will take another three to four decades for graduating classes to see for themselves what the donation of organs portends for the future and the extraordinary benefits that transplantation will provide.

The most successful donation programs are those that include a nurse, chaplain or social worker who has been trained to approach the grieving family with tact and sensitivity. At our hospital the nurse or social worker frequently raises the question of organ donation. A nurse can sometimes succeed in reaching an agreement with a family more readily than a physician could. This is because the family is often more acquainted with the nurse, who is constantly at the patient's bedside. Because a great deal of trust is built by day-to-day contact between nurses and families, it is very important for nurses to be trained in the process of organ donation and how to discuss it with families.

At present, most medical schools and nursing programs do not include courses in the transplantation and donation of organs. Just as doctors and nurses are taught how to help a grieving family and how to promote preventative health care, so also should curricula feature the skills needed to broach the subject of organ donation in a professional, sensitive and purposeful way.

The benefits of organ transplants must be emphasized in hospitals and in professional educational programs, and hospitals must adopt guidelines and set up an audit to ensure compliance. Most physicians graduated before AIDS was even heard of. But the reality of this threat to society has compelled physicians to learn about the AIDS virus. This should also be the case for organ transplantation.

An explicit donation policy within a hospital can have a major educational impact on staff. In hospitals with dialysis programs, the medical and administrative staff are usually sensitized to the desperate need for kidney transplants. They witness patients being hooked up to dialysis machines to have their blood cleansed. It is not surprising that 93 percent of hospitals with dialysis programs have formulated policies that encourage organ donation, while only 36 percent of hospitals with no dialysis units have formulated such policies.

Right now, less than half of all hospitals in Canada have an organ donation policy to promote organ donation. In 1986, in hospitals of 400 beds or more in Canada, 85 percent of car accident victims who died did not have their organs made available for transplants. Why? Because most physicians did not approach the families to ask for donations.

It will take time for attending physicians, medical support staff and the scientific community to recognize the incredible opportunities to save lives and to minimize costs by means of organ transplants that reduce the number of people languishing in hospitals, just waiting to die.

ORGANS AND THE ESSENCE OF LIFE

In a pluralistic society, it is difficult for the attending doctor to know the best approach to take when dealing with a grieving family. Given the many religious viewpoints encountered in the western world, it is important for medical personnel to develop some basic questions that can guide a discussion with the family. Patients and family members do not usually care whether their doctor has the same religious views as they do. But they do expect consideration and respect for their personal beliefs about life, death and the use of organs.

While the topic of what constitutes the "essence of life" may seem philosophical and beyond the scope of a doctor's usual conversation, it is not enough for a doctor or nurse to leave the subject of the spiritual to a rabbi, minister or priest. Family members will want the opinion of a medical professional. Some will ask: "Has the spirit left the body?"

Because, traditionally, physicians have linked the notion of a person's spirit with evidence of physical life, it goes against the grain of our experience to take organs from the body that held the "essence" of a person. There is a wide range of ideas as to what constitutes the essence of a person. As physicians, we struggle to define the existence of the human and find it very difficult to separate the qualitative aspect (the personality and the spirit or soul of the person) from the quantitative aspect (the physical life of the person). In qualitative terms, when a patient experiences brain death, life ceases. Yet quantitatively, physical life continues as long as the body is kept on a respirator.

It is by the qualitative aspects that a person is remembered. Those are the key elements that friends and relatives are concerned about. Relatives usually receive comfort in knowing that the person really has died and is no longer living even though the body continues to function on a respirator. One can see the sense of relief when they finally grasp the fact that the life they see in the body maintained by a life-support system is no longer life from the standpoint of the person they once knew. The functioning of the organs is only mechanical.

In my experience, medical personnel who have yet to come to terms with their own personal views on life and death are the most uncomfortable with this discussion. A physician's lack of understanding in the realm of personhood or the soul becomes quite evident when this understanding is most needed to comfort a family in crisis.

TIMING

Asking for an organ donation is a delicate task in which timing is all-important. The appropriate procedure should work like this: When patients are first admitted to hospital, they are there for the sole purpose of having their lives saved. *There should be no mention of organ donation at that time.* While the patient is receiving active treatment, the family is interested in survival, not organ donation.

Transplantation should not be referred to prior to a pronouncement of brain death. However, when the medical team recognizes the inevitability of brain death in a patient, it is appropriate to inform staff in the intensive care unit and others who might be involved in organ transplants in the event that brain death is declared.

Once a declaration of brain death has been made by the physicians independent of the transplant team, the question of organ donation can be discussed with the relatives.

I was once called to emergency to talk to a family about the possibility of making an organ donation. A neurology resident and an emergency room physician had asked me to visit the family, who were in terrible shock at the sudden death of a loved one. As I entered the room, I could feel tension and the family avoided eye contact with me. They answered my questions with tight-lipped expressions and clipped sentences.

I decided to face the hostility head-on. I asked, as kindly as I could, why they were reacting to me in the way they were. I made it clear that I did not want to add to their sorrow by talking about organ donation.

A distraught woman explained that when her sister had been wheeled into emergency and was examined, the question of organ donation had been raised. The woman then asked if they could be referred to another hospital where the staff was more interested in caring for patients than in finding organ donors. When asked later if they would agree to donate the organs of their loved one, the family refused. Their decision was irrevocable, and all because the subject was raised at the wrong time. Health care teams must be aware of the family's extreme sensitivity to the needs of the dying relative, and staff must try to get the timing right.

CRITICAL STEPS IN OBTAINING A DONOR

I want to outline the steps an attending physician should take in encouraging an organ donation. While this information is obviously intended for doctors, I include it here so everyone has a better understanding of what to expect.

Step 1
The attending physician realizes that the patient is, or will be, a potential donor as a result of anticipated brain death. A neurological examination demonstrates whether brain stem reflexes are absent. The exam verifies whether or not brain death has occurred.

Step 2
The physician determines that the patient is not a victim of cancer, hepatitis or AIDS.

Step 3
The attending physician should conduct an examination of the patient for signs of brain death and officially record that brain death has occurred. A second physician's opinion is also required.

Step 4
The physician phones the local organ retrieval service and asks to speak to the coordinator responsible for organ donations. If a message is left, the coordinator should return the call within minutes of being notified about a potential donor. In the course of a telephone consultation the doctor and the coordinator can assess the need for organs.

If no local organ retrieval service exists, the regional, provincial or state retrieval center should be notified immediately. These telephone numbers should be posted conspicuously in every intensive care unit and emergency department.

Step 5
The attending physician and the transplant coordinator discuss which organs can be retrieved from the patient.

Step 6
The attending physician, nurse or social worker approaches the family, preferably in a face-to-face meeting. The discussion should include several topics about which the family will need specific answers. The physician must spend enough time with the family so they feel that none of their questions has been overlooked or considered irrelevant.

The doctor should explain that, following the declaration of brain death, the donor will remain in the ICU for a few hours while arrangements are made for the retrieval team to reach the hospital. In some cases, the donor's body may be transferred to another hospital. If so, this will take extra time and the family of the donor should be given all details so they don't develop the feeling that medical personnel are keeping something from them.

The family's questions should be anticipated and met with specific answers. Here are some common questions:

(a) *Who decides if there is brain death?*
The family must be assured that the diagnosis of brain death has been made, or will be made, by two physicians who are not associated with the organ retrieval team. Also, it should be made clear that the diagnosis of brain death will be based on clinical criteria. Explain whether or not brain tracing (EEG) or a study of brain blood flow will be done.

(b) *Is there a chance of a mistake?*
Assure the family that the diagnosis of brain death is definitive and that if the criteria are met, there is no possibility of error.

The doctor should comment on the discrepancy between what seems to be no change in the bodily appearance of the donor and brain death. This is often difficult to accept emotionally, not only by the relatives but also by members of the health care team. The patient continues to have a good heartbeat with normal blood pressure and the skin is warm to the touch. However, the patient is dead because the brain is no longer functioning. The family may need time to accept the finality of the diagnosis of brain death before the next step is taken.

If the family wishes to have an independent consultation with a neurologist or a neurosurgeon, this should be arranged either in person, or, if a specialist is not available in your community, by telephone. A consultation service is also available through the regional retrieval center.

(c) *How will the donor's body be handled?*
Explain to the family that the body will be taken to the operating room with the life-support systems still intact and that the same degree of respect that was given to the patient in life will be given in death. The organs will be removed with a recognition that the precious "substance of life" is being transferred from one human being to another. At no time will the body be scarred in a way that would interfere with public viewing at a funeral home.

(d) *Which organs will be used?*
While attending physicians may not always agree with the wishes of the family, they should always respect the relatives' decision regarding the organs they want to donate. These wishes should be absolutely adhered to. The family's decision should be obtained during a second conversation following the meeting when the concept of donation was first introduced.

In my experience, I have found it important to reassure the family that the primary concern is to restore someone's life — not to use organs for research. The family should be assured that any organ taken will be used, except, of course, if certain serious diseases that were not detected prior to death make the organ unuseable.

Step 7
The physician should notify the retrieval service that written consent has been obtained from the family. The retrieval service will schedule when the team or teams should move the patient to the operating room. If lungs or heart and lungs are being

donated, the donor may need to be transferred to another hospital by ambulance or air ambulance because lungs must be transplanted within a very short time. The family's consent must be obtained before such a move can be made.

Step 8
The physician should gently advise the family to return home, assuring them that they will be informed when everything has been completed and the body of their loved one has been sent to the morgue. In two to three weeks, the family will receive a letter from the organ retrieval center telling them which organs were used and providing a general description of the recipients. Although the donor's family sometimes learns who received the organ, in Canada the Human Tissue Gift Act protects this information. This guarantees the anonymity of both donor and recipient and prevents any potential conflict.

Step 9
The organ retrieval service is responsible for booking the operating room, arranging transportation and finalizing details with the coroner.

Step 10
Finally, there is the flurry of surgical activity. The medical team will retrieve and pack the various organs and move on to the second phase of their journey of hope.

When all is quiet, the attending physician can feel satisfied that through the family's generosity:

- a young woman will awaken from an anesthetic with a healthy new heart;
- a young man will awaken from a coma with a healthy new liver;
- a dying father will breathe with new lungs and will return home to his family;
- a mother will receive a new kidney that will free her from the prison of dialysis;

- two blind people will see; and
- a severely burned child will stabilize as her body cover is restored.

Believe me when I say that there is no experience in medicine that surpasses the satisfaction of being involved with this transfer of life from one human being to another.

WHO GIVES?

THERE IS A WIDESPREAD presumption that people are reluctant to donate their organs or those of their next of kin. This is simply not true. On the contrary, people have an enormous desire and capacity to give. Where organ donation is concerned, the need is to inform rather than to persuade the public.

It took a media event to shock Canadians into taking notice of the lack of donors. In 1985, Ike Brydlt, a successful business-man in Edmonton, Alberta who had been on dialysis for years because of kidney failure, openly solicited a donor kidney.

Despite his illness, Ike kept his business going, maintained his family life and participated in community activities. But he became increasingly disturbed by what kidney disease was doing to him. Each time he went to the hospital for dialysis, he asked his doctor if a donor kidney had been found. Each time the doctor responded that no suitable match had been found.

Ike knew that at that time 90 percent of all potential kidney donations were being wasted. The reason? Few people were being asked to donate. Although there were many available kidneys, which with a little effort could have been donated, Ike's life continued to be compromised. He got angry and took matters into his own hands. He reasoned that if certain people could donate a kidney to a relative with little risk to themselves, why couldn't someone who wasn't a relative do the same? He put an ad in the local paper offering $5,000 (Canadian) to anyone who would sell him a kidney.

Reaction was instantaneous. Radio, television and newspapers ran the story and it became headline news. Journalists rained criticism and scorn on Ike. "How could he put a dollar value on human life?" they asked. "How could a person offer money for human tissue?"

Hundreds responded to Ike's newspaper ad. The media continued to run the story, intrigued by how many people were prepared to sell a part of their body. However, journalists overlooked one of the most vital aspects of the story: 85 percent of those who responded said they were not interested in money. They simply wanted to help Ike. The media ignored this fact. For cynics, this was a story about people trying to make a fast buck. While it is true that many people responded for that reason alone, the press failed to acknowledge the altruism of those 85 percent who were willing to undergo personal risk for someone in need. These people responded not out of crass materialism, but because donating an organ seemed a small price to pay to bring someone else health and freedom. Ike eventually received a cadaveric organ, and lived.

In my experiences, there is a growing desire among people to participate in both the giving and the restoring of life. The perception within the medical community that the main barrier to increased organ donation is the reluctance of individuals or families to give is absolutely false.

A Gallup poll conducted in the United States and reported in the *New York Times* in May, 1987, posed the question: "Would you agree to donate the organs of your adult relatives after death?" Eighty-two percent of respondents said "yes," and 61 percent said they would give their permission if it were their child. When asked if they would donate their own organs, 48 percent said "yes." But when asked if they had signed an organ donor card, only 20 percent said they had.

In 1984 an Ontario government task force survey asked, "Would you agree to the donation of your relative's organs if you were asked after brain death had been declared?" Eighty-eight percent of respondents said they would. In the same survey, 63 percent said they wished to donate their own organs, but only 25 percent had signed a donor consent card.

I know from my own experience that when people have been properly informed about organ donation by a physician, nurse, social worker or the clergy, only a small percentage refuse.

DONOR CARDS OF CONSENT

In North America, the primary method of recording the wish to donate an organ is to sign an organ donor card, usually located on the back of a driver's license. Alternatively, in some jurisdictions a signed donor card can be carried in a wallet or purse. The organ donor card system was devised on the premise that individuals are entitled to donate their organs after death if they so wish. The system was developed in the mid-1970s when organ transplants became more common and governments began to encourage the public to donate. As people were alerted to the urgent need for organs, these documents were made readily accessible in some jurisdictions, so physicians could quickly determine a person's written consent to remove organs for transplant.

The most obvious challenge in making this system work is getting people to sign the consent card. Doctors typically discover, however, that in 75 percent of cases the person has not signed the consent card.

Some people conclude that because of the low success rate in persuading drivers to sign a donor card (the percentages vary between 7 to 27 percent, depending on the region) the public is reluctant to give. In reviewing the Canadian Gallup poll, 1983, it is my view that the low percentage of signing reflects a psychological block; people fail to sign a form that is linked to the possibility of their own death. Most people shy away from contemplating death and making decisions related to it.

In an Ontario survey, we asked: In the event that people had signed their organ donor card permitting organ donation in case of death, would they be willing to allow their relatives the right to override that decision and refuse organ donation? All respondents insisted that the donor card should be treated as a legal document and not disputed by the next of kin.

The second challenge in making the signed consent forms really work is getting the document to the right place at the right time. If death is caused by a traffic accident, for example, police may keep the driver's license for their investigation. When the victim's body arrives at the hospital, the signed organ donation card is therefore missing and hospital staff cannot determine the deceased's wishes concerning transplants.

To complicate matters, the medical profession is reluctant to test the donor card system in the courts. Even though the Human Tissue Gift Act has been legislated in all Canadian provinces (except in Quebec where it is covered under the Quebec Civil Code) we don't know whether the signed documents will stand up in court. While the Human Tissue Gift Act states unequivocally that the physician or surgeon has the right to use the organ donor card as signed by the donor and does not have to refer to the next of kin, it is unlikely that a doctor would override the wishes of relatives and act on the basis of a previously signed card.

In the United States, the Uniform Anatomical Gift Act (1987) has been approved for enactment in all states. But there, as in Canada, its legality has not been tested.

This problem will be resolved only when the public refuses to allow the medical profession to use as an excuse the small percentage of citizens who sign an organ donor card. Among those who die each year, 25 percent have signed a card and yet only 12 percent of these become sources of organ donations. Again, failure results because doctors either do not check to see if the victim has signed a consent form, or they do not approach the relatives for permission to have organs donated.

What will it take to overcome this failure? As the public becomes more proactive with respect to organ donations and better informed about the shortage of available organs, the medical and hospital systems will be pressured to change their attitudes. Indeed, the momentum generated by public demand may push doctors to ensure that organ donations become much more common in a hospital. And perhaps hospital boards will insist upon an explicit policy to ensure that organs are not needlessly wasted.

Another solution lies in having doctors and nurses realize that relatives are not hindrances but facilitators in the process. The medical profession must appreciate the benefits that a family gains when they agree to donate organs. The process of donating the organs of a loved one who has just been declared dead unquestionably helps alleviate a family's sorrow and loss.

ALTERNATIVE DONOR PLANS

Within the medical profession, an internal plan is needed to ensure that every opportunity for organ donation is taken. An administrative procedure called "recorded consideration" is a medical audit system that checks whether organs from all patients who die in a hospital have been retrieved, and why or why not. In this system, a physician is required to record the following data on a chart:

1. Was the patient a potential donor?
   Yes or no. If no, why not?

2. Were the relatives asked about organ donations?
   Yes or no. If no, why not?

3. What was the outcome?
   Which organs were donated?

Some state legislatures in the United States have implemented a procedure called "required request." This goes beyond "recorded consideration" by requiring that physicians not only monitor organ retrieval but also approach the next of kin regarding organ donation. This system requires the hospital to follow the procedure or lose financial reimbursement for patient care.

Some countries have a system called "presumed consent." This system presumes that individuals are willing to be organ donors unless they have signed a card stating otherwise. This places the responsibility on each person to say "no" to having their organs donated if that is their choice. If people haven't signed a card to indicate their wishes, then the health care system presumes that they have agreed to donate their organs.

If the Canadian government passed laws instituting "presumed consent," I would actively oppose it. I have seen too many families cope with grief and self-pity through genuine giving; I could not rob them of the opportunity to make this choice themselves.

The ultimate arrogance is to propose a system of "mandatory consent." In such a system the physician is given the right to remove any or all organs after death. This is hardly a solution.

As medical practitioners, we must urge the public to sign their donor cards and inform their relatives of their wishes. And furthermore, we must congratulate them for doing so. Eventually, the public will exert pressure on the medical community, forcing them to pay much more attention to the simple but critical act of signing donor consent cards. Public expectation combined with improved medical procedures will ultimately produce an abundant supply of organs for transplant.

USE AND MISUSE
OF THE MEDIA

I T WAS A SLOW NIGHT in a downtown Toronto newsroom. The only sounds were the strident voices from equipment monitoring calls from the police, fire department and ambulance services.

Suddenly, a weary reporter snapped to attention as she heard the following on a police radio: "Attention, units in the vicinity of Highways 427 and 401. Toronto Western Hospital is doing a heart transplant. They need police escorts to get them to the airport. Cars that are free in 15 minutes, please check in."

The reporter learned that a team of surgeons would soon be flying by chartered jet from Toronto to London, where a young male car accident victim was being sustained on a respirator at the University Hospital.

The same message was heard in other newspaper, radio and television newsrooms in that part of the province, and soon a dozen eager reporters were rushing to find out all they could. Telephone calls deluged transplant officials at the Toronto and London hospitals. Within hours, the transplant had taken place, the family of the young man in London had arranged a funeral, and the family of the recipient in Toronto had reason to rejoice.

With the exception of AIDS, organ transplants have attracted more attention from the media than any other medical story. Even though multiple-organ transplants are becoming increasingly common, keen interest in the subject has not waned among journalists and broadcasters. This interest on the part of the media is vitally important. When an extraordinary medical event happens, the attention focused on it by the press helps to disseminate information and raise awareness of the urgent need for more donor organs. Every time a story about an organ transplant reaches the public, it serves to highlight that there are people on waiting lists who will die unless a donor is located. Often journalists run a story not just because it is good copy, but because they truly want to help, by reaching and influencing a large number of people.

PROBLEMS WITH THE MEDIA

Along with some of my medical colleagues, I have been accused of using or manipulating the media. At first this accusation offended me, but on closer examination I realized it may be true. There are times when our medical team is desperate to help a patient who will die if an organ donor is not found. In our frustration over the lack of response to this dilemma and in an effort to get the public to sit up and take notice, we sometimes go directly to the press.

However, the recruiting of organs for specific recipients through media channels is particularly problematic. On a segment of "The Donahue Show" recorded in New York City in June 1986 a direct appeal was made for a heart to save a dying child. A family who had seen the program came forward and offered the heart of their child, who was dying in an ICU. The implication of the result of this media appeal was that, in future, the family having the best access to the public through the media would be most likely to get a transplant first. The child lived as a result of the appeal.

Using the media to appeal for donors has both a positive and a negative side. On the one hand, it creates a greater awareness of the need for organ donations. On the other hand, it suggests that the best way for a family to find an organ is to solicit the assistance of the media in "campaigning" for a donor.

The negative fallout from publicity-seeking is higher in the United States than in Canada, for one essential reason. In the U.S., even if a donor is found, money immediately becomes an issue. If the recipient's family does not have adequate insurance coverage, they are required in most instances by the hospital to prove that they can pay for transplant costs. And in the case of a liver transplant, the cost, in 1988, was a minimum $100,000, which did not include physician's fees, transportation costs or outpatient aftercare expenses! In Canada, all patients, regardless of economic status, are covered by Provincial medical insurance.

When these two powerful institutions — the medical establishment and the media — come into close contact, there is a danger of misunderstanding. Seeing the enormous good they can effect, the media run stories to capture the public imagination, and, in the process, increase awareness of the need for donors. Many doctors, however, are inclined to privacy and may regard the stories as an invasion of their territory. Some doctors react cynically, assuming that the media's real interest is to enhance ratings and circulation. This reaction, in turn, may cause reporters to be less cordial or sensitive in their treatment of the subject.

The medical profession must realize that the media, in order to be effective, must have a *concrete* story. It is one thing to write about the need for people to sign their donor cards and to exert pressure on the medical community to be more proactive in organ solicitation. It is difficult, though, for journalists to explain the problem of organ transplants unless they have a specific story to hang it on.

Also, both journalists and the public are interested in human drama, especially if a story is a local one. If a person in need of a transplant — especially a child — lives in the community, there is more interest and concern about that person's needs, compared to someone halfway across the continent. Neither may there be much interest in an abstract explanation of how a waiting list works. Thus, the compelling need of a local child who is in critical need of an organ transplant supersedes a story concerning the general need for organ donations. A television camera is much more drawn to the tears of the dying child's mother than to the dry subject of administrative systems. The electronic and print media are oriented towards real-life drama. And the medical community cannot expect it to shift its orientation.

One initiative has helped to resolve the chaos of "line-jumping" and questions of "who gets the organ?", issues that peaked in the mid-1980s. This important initiative has been the establishment of a rating system and of waiting lists. (For details, see Chapter 4.) The list has effectively eliminated the possibility of queue-jumping. Even if a family goes public in their search for an organ, they will not receive an organ if they do not meet the necessary medical criteria. Also, media personnel have become increasingly sophisticated in their understanding of medical information and procedures. Many networks and newspapers refuse to run stories unless they are convinced that the story is bona fide and supported by the organ distribution system.

There is a danger, however, that a family frustrated by what they perceive as inertia may bypass their doctor and the system and go directly to the media, expecting that reporters will beat a path to their door. If the media refuse to cooperate because they haven't received clearance from the medical community, the family may feel discriminated against and hostility towards their doctor may be intensified. Families must try to understand that just because certain cases are noticed by the media does not mean that every need for an organ transplant will be automatically promoted on TV or in the press.

Hospitals are always in dire need of public donations to help finance equipment purchases and operational expenses. A danger lurks that a hospital will decide to branch into organ transplants because of the opportunity to attract public interest and thus enhance their financial appeals. It might be assumed that if an organ transplant unit is set up, the hospital will become better known and will receive more funds from foundations and individuals.

The real issue is not whether going public is valid (which I believe it is). Rather, it is whether the need to involve the media has been exploited in order to raise a hospital's profile as a means of increasing its budget. If so, both the media and the public are being manipulated. There is a fine line between manipulation and legitimate servicing.

The press sometimes has unrealistic expectations of the medical community. In exchange for their cooperation media personnel may try to find out the name and age of the donor or the city from which the donor organ came. Under the Human Tissue Gift Act in Canada (see Appendix D), it is illegal for a physician to reveal this information. While some people in the media might not appreciate this, it is essential to preserve anonymity.

Often, of course, recipient families find out who the donor is and sometimes this information leaks out to the press. Sometimes aggressive reporters dig up the information and use it in print or on the air. In January of 1988, for example, a newspaper in Nashville, Tennessee ran the headline: "Heart-Lung Transplant Underway." In this case, however, the donor had committed suicide. Her mother was employed at the medical institution that performed the transplant. In subsequent editions that followed up on the story, the name and address of the girl and her mother were revealed, along with personal details such as the mother's previous loss of employment and divorce. This coverage represented a terrible breach of trust.

SUCCESSFUL INTERVENTION BY THE MEDIA

In general, I have found reporters and broadcasters to be not only responsible, but also deeply committed to helping in any way they can. The most dramatic example of this commitment occurred at our center in 1986.

In August of that year, four-year-old Gabriel Bruce, who lived with his grandparents on an Indian Reserve in northern Manitoba, was admitted to a Winnipeg hospital with a mysterious liver ailment, later diagnosed as a type of hepatitis. After two weeks the little boy's condition worsened and he was transferred to the University Hospital in London. Gabriel had developed jaundice and was suffering from internal and external bleeding, as well as breathing difficulties. His belly was distended. One reporter from the *London Free Press* observed that he looked like a starving child in a famine-stricken country.

Because Gabriel's liver had been destroyed by a virus, his condition deteriorated rapidly. Dr. Morris Jenner, medical coordinator of the Joint Pediatric Transplant Unit at University Hospital and the Children's Hospital of Western Ontario in London, told me that he thought the four-year-old could go into a coma at any time and that if nothing were done, he would be dead within a week.

Like the other doctors caring for him, I knew Gabriel was extremely susceptible to an infection, and that we were running out of time. I decided that the only means of saving his life was an immediate liver transplant.

Because Gabriel's situation was an emergency, we decided to go public. I talked it over with the other doctors and we realized we would be open to criticism. But a child's life was at stake, and we had tried the conventional route — the donor network — without success.

My colleagues and I called a press conference at the boy's bedside. Gabriel's grandmother collapsed in tears into the arms of a nurse while her usually stoic husband buried his head in a pillow to hide his despair. The media attention that was focused on the little boy was almost more than the family could bear.

Although we were convinced that we had done the right thing, we received a lot of flak. We were bombarded with criticism, ranging from "Should this little boy be the next on the list just because of all the publicity?" to "They are exploiting this little boy to arouse public sympathy because he is a native Canadian Indian."

Within our computerized rating system, Gabriel was a status 6, the highest-priority rating for a recipient at that time. This meant he would be the next recipient of a donated liver unless we learned of another child even more ill than Gabriel.

I felt that our medical team was acting as an honest advocate for Gabriel's family. However, our decision to help also brought confusion and distress to the family. They experienced culture shock as they were thrust into a high-tech environment and became the focus of a media event. They were distracted by cameras, tape recorders and notepads documenting their every word and tear.

The criticism of our decision to go public was widespread. One reporter asked me if I thought it was appropriate to circumvent the system to help one specific patient. The question angered me. I responded with an analogy: Suppose someone were trapped on the sixth floor of a burning building. The person leans out the window and yells for help, in one last desperate attempt to be saved. But someone below responds, "Don't shout, we have a system in place. It's called the fire department and a call has been put in. So don't worry — wait for the system to work and stop shouting!"

As the days passed, the media focused more and more on how desperate the situation had become. As journalists researched the subject of organ transplants, they became more knowledgeable and articulate, with regard to both surgery and the immune system. Dozens of calls from well-wishers flooded in. Then Gabriel took a turn for the worse. Everyone despaired that help would arrive in time. However, Dr. Tim Frewen, chief of the pediatric critical care unit, announced that Gabriel's condition had stabilized and that the boy was in good spirits.

The most frustrating aspect of this case was that we knew somewhere, in some hospital on the continent, there had to be a potential donor, a child whose life was being sustained by a respirator. David Grant, a young surgeon on the transplant team, spoke for us all when he said, "We want to avoid the tragedy of an individual dying while waiting for an organ. Especially since we know that nine out of ten organs that could potentially be used in a transplant are not offered for organ donation."

On September 19, we held the opening ceremonies for the John P. Robarts Research Institute at the University Hospital in London. One of the guests was the Honorable Jake Epp, then Minister of Health and Welfare for Canada. Knowing of his interest in transplants, I prevailed on Mr. Epp and his wife Lydia to join me in a visit to Gabriel's bedside in the pediatric critical care unit. Later that day the minister sought out the media with an impassioned appeal for help. But there was no response.

Finally, after a barrage of media coverage and public appeals made across Canada and the United States, the wheels were set in motion. Two physicians in Joplin, Missouri, Dr. Hish Majzoub and Dr. Kurt Dandridge, heard a news story about the desperate race to save a child's life in London, Ontario. They asked the parents of another little boy who had died if they would consider donation. The parents agreed. Dr. Bill Wall, head of liver transplantation, and Dr. John Duff, chief of surgery, performed the transplant later that night.

Once the transplant had been performed, Gabriel improved almost immediately. The jaundice, swelling and bleeding cleared up. Shortly after emerging from the operating room, Gabriel awoke and recognized the family members at his bedside. There was an avalanche of cards and gifts from people all over the country. School children wrote messages of encouragement. The media reported every change in his condition and followed his recovery vigilantly.

A year later, a *London Free Press* reporter, Dahlia Reich, visited Winnipeg to follow up on the story. She found Gabriel happy and healthy. Concerns about the poor living conditions that physicians thought might interfere with his recovery were nullified. Native Family Support Services had furnished a three-bedroom home for Gabriel and his grandparents. The family had pulled together and Gabriel was thriving.

This event in transplant history was a double triumph. One child's death had at least given another child life. Also, the public had learned more about the need for donor organs and the process of transplantation than ever before.

As new advances are made in transplantation, I expect that the media will continue to demonstrate great interest. For this we are grateful. While protecting the privacy of patients and donor families, we nevertheless have an obligation to remind the public at every opportunity that Canadians are dying, not because we lack medical knowledge, but because we have too few donors.

We know that in the future transplants will lose their novelty. Also, the problems of diseased and AIDS-infected organs, the normal failure rate and the issue of "organs for sale" will cause reporters and journalists to become less enamored of transplants, so that the negative aspects will receive more publicity. Even then, however, the public will at least become more knowledgeable.

LIVING DONATIONS

WHEN SUCCESSFUL TRANSPLANTATION began in the early 1950s, doctors discovered that kidney transplants between identical twins had a high rate of success and did not require agents to suppress the immune response. Since that time, "living donation" between relatives has constituted about 20 percent of all kidney transplants. No other organ, with the exceptions of bone marrow and liver, has a similar potential. A lung could not be donated, for example, because of the risk to the donor. However, it is possible to live on only one kidney, and a donor's bone marrow can replenish itself.

SIBLING DONORS

Myrna (not real name), a 31-year-old woman from a farming community, suffered from chronic kidney failure and had been on dialysis for three years. She was married, with no children. Her husband, who was often unemployed, was not emotionally supportive. When Myrna became ill and required dialysis, however, he took on a full-time job.

Myrna's illness was evident in her sallow, yellow skin, her increasingly fine hair and her rippled fingernails, all symptoms of kidney failure. Although she never complained, from time to time she said how wonderful it would be if she no longer had to be hooked up to a machine for six hours a day, three days a week.

Each time, she would leave the dialysis unit feeling unwell, facing a long drive home. She had been on a waiting list for a new kidney for almost two years.

Finally, Myrna's two sisters and two brothers decided to talk to me about becoming donors themselves. I met with them to explain the process. I said that although we are born with two kidneys, if one kidney is removed at an early age due to disease, or if an accident destroys one kidney, there is no evidence that life expectancy is therefore reduced.

In fact, the results of living donations of kidneys have been so good that insurance companies require no extra premium for someone who has made a living donation, and they show no hesitation in insuring those having only one kidney.

Giving a kidney to a relative or loved one is an incredible sacrifice. It means undergoing pain and anxiety, and enduring a stay in hospital. While employment benefits may cover the financial costs of being off work, the personal costs — pain and disruption of one's life — must also be considered. It is not a decision to be taken lightly.

I told Myrna's family that if one or more of the siblings chose to donate, extensive testing would be required. Also, the major surgery involved would leave a large scar. More importantly, I reminded them there is some risk associated with the procedure. It has been calculated that the mortality risk to a living kidney donor is equivalent to driving 2.5 km (1.5 miles) farther to work in a North American city every day.

I explained that within a family the donor and recipient must have compatible blood groups, and that the best results occur when two individuals are identical by tissue type. When an organ is transplanted from one person to another (described in Chapter 2), the body recognizes the difference between self and the new organ. The tissue type that the body recognizes as self is determined by genetic characteristics inherited from the father and mother. These genetic characteristics, called the "major histocompatibility complex" or "HLA," are located on the sixth chromosome. When the egg divides and unites with the sperm, the child receives half the genetic information from the mother and half from the father. This leads to four possible combinations of this genetic information: a or b from the mother, and c or d from the father.

Child number 1 — the ac child — receives the a tissue type from the mother and the c tissue type from the father. The second child — the ad child — receives the a type from the mother and the d type from the father. Likewise, child number 3 — the bc child — receives the b type from the mother and the c type from the father. The fourth possibility, the only remaining one, is that the fourth child — the bd child — receives the b type from the mother and the d type from the father. Any other child is identical to one of these four: ac, bc, ad, or bd.

If a transplant is done between child ac and bd, it is as though child bd has received a kidney from someone completely unrelated. The reason for this is that the two children do not have a similar genetic "package" of information from their father and

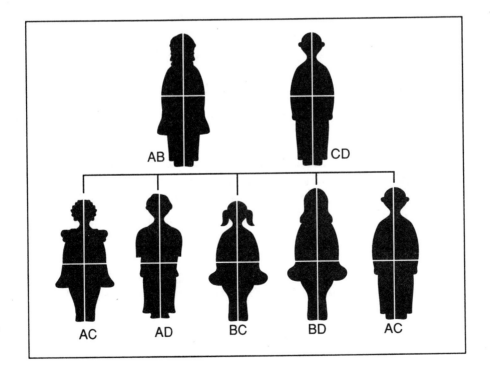

mother, and are therefore completely nonidentical in terms of their tissue types.

On the other hand, if child ac receives a kidney from child ad, half the genetic information — c and d — is different, but the half that they have obtained from the mother is identical. Both children have received the a genetic information from the mother. In this case, the immune system would be challenged by only half the degree of dissimilarity that the first donor-recipient combination gave, so that the results, in terms of chances of rejection, are considerably improved. The statistical difference in results between these two combinations is about 10 percent. In other words, the first combination, ac and bd, would have a success rate of about 80 percent. The second combination — ac transplanted to ad or bc — would have a success rate of approximately 90 percent.

The ideal transplant, of course, is between two siblings who have exactly the same genetic makeup, for example, an ac transplanted to an ac; in such cases, the success rate is almost 100 percent. This is almost like doing a transplant between identical twins. The minor differences in the tissue match require only a small dosage of immunosuppressive drugs to inhibit rejection. (The only time that antirejection drugs are not used is in an organ transplant between identical twins.) The drug dosage is directly related to the degree of difference in the tissue match. The greater the difference, the greater the drug dosage required.

After I had explained these genetic factors to Myrna's family, I said, "We don't know which one of you is identical, half identical or not identical at all. We won't know until we've tissue-typed all of you. I want to make it very clear that I don't want any of you to feel you have to give. I know you are here because you are concerned about your sister and you want the best for her. But some of you may feel very fearful of this operation and therefore not be able to go through with it. Others may be prepared to face it."

I have found that the testing and selection process can be

either unifying or disruptive for the family. Therefore, I told them that, to protect the integrity of the family, I would tissue-type each sibling and report only individual results to each person.

"In addition," I said, "I'll ask you to see our social worker, June Burley [at that time our social worker for kidney patients], and our psychiatrist, Dr. Mai. They will talk to you about your private fears and concerns and the impact that donation might have on your life and that of your family. You can then decide privately what you want to do. Nothing you discuss will be transmitted to other members of the family or to your sister. In the final analysis, of course, a medical examination will determine whether you are fit to give a kidney. If you have high blood pressure or the potential for developing diabetes or anything else that might affect the functioning of your kidney, I reserve the right to reject you as a donor on medical grounds.

"Now suppose you are, in fact, medically fit and identical in tissue type to your sister. Nevertheless, if either Dr. Mai or Mrs. Burley advises me that psychological, social or emotional factors would compromise your health if you were to give a kidney, then I will not consider you a candidate for donation."

After a detailed orientation, I arranged for blood to be taken from each of Myrna's siblings for tissue typing and I asked the staff to report the results to me confidentially. We then ordered some basic medical tests for each sibling. We did an x-ray and an ultrasound of each person's kidneys, checked kidney function and screened for any prediabetic symptoms.

Two siblings were nonidentical. One brother shared half his sister's genetic makeup. Unfortunately, Myrna had received blood transfusions and had built up antibodies in her system which in the test showed that her system would probably reject her brother's kidney.

The fourth sibling, Paul, was identical in tissue type to Myrna. He was young and fit. In all respects, he was an ideal donor.

I called the first three family members privately and told them that they were unable to give Myrna a kidney. When Paul came to see me, his wife came with him. I told him that he was identical: his kidney would match perfectly.

The husband's and wife's responses were dramatically different. Paul, who loved his sister dearly, broke into a smile. But his wife's countenance fell. Her mouth tightened and she clutched her hands as she perched on the edge of her chair and glared at her husband.

I asked Paul's wife what she thought. She said, "Dr. Stiller, I understand why Paul wants to give a kidney to Myrna. We both love her. She is a perfect wife and a wonderful sister. But I despise that husband of hers for how he treats her. I have no doubt that as soon as she receives her new kidney and gets off dialysis, he will quit work again. And once more, she'll have to find work to support him."

She paused, then turned to her husband. "Paul, if you get into medical trouble by giving one of your kidneys and you aren't able to work, or if you get sick and die, my children will be robbed of a father and I of a husband I love dearly. I would never be able to handle that."

Paul didn't know what to say. He was torn between his desire to help his sister and the reality that, for his wife, this was an unacceptable option.

I took a gentle approach as we discussed the alternative. We would continue to look for a kidney donated by someone who had died.

I reminded Paul that if his sister received a kidney from a stranger who had died, and five or ten years later the kidney failed, he would have to live with the fact that perhaps his donation would have worked better. However, I told him that I sympathized with him in his dilemma, and that it was up to him to make a decision that would spare both his conscience and his marriage.

I told Paul and his wife that after further tests were performed on Paul, they would have one final opportunity to make their decision.

The test results came in. I called Paul and told him that on the basis of these test results I would have to turn down his offer on medical grounds. He did not ask any questions. I knew he didn't want to hear any more. I then told Myrna that none of her brothers or sisters could be considered potential donors.

About three months later, an acquaintance of mine and his wife were rushing out to a formal dinner. Dressed in a long gown, the woman tripped and tumbled down the basement stairs, striking her head on the concrete floor. She was rushed to the hospital, where she was declared brain-dead.

When I suggested a kidney donation to the woman's husband, he grasped the opportunity and gave his consent. In reviewing the list of those waiting for a transplant, we discovered there was a compatible tissue cross-match with Myrna, which meant increased chances of the kidney surviving the transplant. That night Myrna received a new kidney. She coped well in the postoperative period and was discharged from hospital.

Eight months later, when a rejuvenated Myrna went back to work, her husband did quit his job, just as Myrna's sister-in-law had predicted.

Eventually, Myrna left her husband, remarried and had two children. Today she enjoys a happy life with her new family.

As the situation above illustrates, all stories of living donation within families do not work out. Family members considering such an option must be prepared to encounter unforeseen emotional conflicts and complications.

Another case of mine had completely unexpected repercussions within the family. The patient, Johanna (not real name), had been on dialysis for four years. She had received two transplants from donors who had died but her body had rejected both kidneys and her health was deteriorating.

Before her illness, Johanna had travelled extensively with her husband. Deprived of this enjoyment, she became increasingly depressed. It had never been my practice to push for family donation. But knowing that Johanna had brothers and sisters, I asked her one day if the family had ever discussed organ donation.

She said that they had done so, five years ago. When they had asked what the risk was in donating an organ, the kidney specialist had replied that it was like crossing a highway blindfolded. Although the probability of getting across the road safely was high, you could not predict if or when you might be hit by oncoming traffic. This dramatic visual image had frightened the family, deterring them from further considering the option of living donation.

I asked if I might talk to the family. Of the eight siblings, five came to see me. Just as I had done with Myrna's family, I explained the benefits and risks of organ donation. This time the siblings agreed to tissue typing. One of the brothers, Gerald, was identical to Johanna. A businessman and the father of several children, Gerald had not had a close relationship with either Johanna or her husband. Gerald came to my office to receive the test results. I told him that he was not only identically matched to his sister, but also he was physically fit and there was no reason for rejecting him on medical grounds.

He responded, "Dr. Stiller, I want to donate, but I want to make clear to you and everyone else that I am donating simply because my sister is a person who needs help. I am not donating because she is my sister. I have not had a close relationship with her and I don't like her husband. I am simply prepared to donate because she needs a kidney. I would do it for anyone in the community."

I discussed Gerald's attitude with the medical team. We believed that his response was genuine and we decided to go ahead with the transplant.

Within seven days Gerald was out of hospital, and in three weeks he had returned to work. The kidney that Johanna had received from her brother functioned immediately and her health blossomed. Her hemoglobin and blood pressure normalized and she was filled with vibrant energy.

Before the operation, Johanna's husband had promised Gerald that he would pay any expenses and, should Gerald develop medical complications or die, he pledged to support his family.

I watched a bond of love and friendship grow within Johanna's family. A brother and sister who had been estranged for years became intimate friends, and Gerald later told me that this had been the most wonderful experience of his life. He had given selflessly, but he had also received, in the form of an extraordinary reunion with his sister. Eight years later, both of them remain well, happy and the best of friends.

EMOTIONALLY RELATED DONORS

For years I have been troubled by situations in which the spouse of a patient on dialysis is willing to give a kidney, but is turned down because the couple is not related by birth. In reality, however, if a kidney cannot be found, then often a spouse *could* serve effectively as a donor.

The idea of an unrelated individual donating a kidney has been frowned upon within the transplant community, because of the possibility that the person is donating for money or out of some form of coercion, such as payment of a debt. This concern dates back to the early days of transplantation in Denver, Colorado, when inmates at the state prison donated kidneys with the suspected motive of receiving better treatment by the parole board, though this was never proven. While I believe that the highest ethical standards prevailed in Denver, the potential for emotional coercion nevertheless existed. But then, the possibility for coercion exists within a family as well.

In my opinion, a husband or wife who wants to donate an organ is more than likely motivated by altruism and love. In studying this dilemma, June Burley and I published an article to assist doctors, psychologists and social workers to deal with both family related and emotionally related donors. June and I both believe that from a psychological standpoint, emotionally related donors are sometimes better donors than blood-related ones.

The Council of the Transplantation Society in 1985 published guidelines which specified that the living, unrelated donor's physician must not be associated with the transplant team or the recipient's physician, to help protect the interests of the donor. These guidelines included later in this chapter are honored worldwide by members of the Transplantation Society, which is made up of physicians who are engaged in organ transplants. And while the results of these guidelines cannot be verified by statistics, their widespread acceptance demonstrates their value.

BUYING AND SELLING ORGANS

A farmer from a nearby community called me one day and asked if he could donate a kidney. I asked him why he wanted to. He said he had recently met someone who was on dialysis and that he had seen a TV special about the need for kidneys. He told me he was 48 yers old, a bachelor without children and financially secure. He simply wished to do something good for humanity. He did not want to know the name of the recipient and he desired no money or public acknowledgment. He simply wanted to donate a kidney.

I frequently receive phone calls or letters from individuals who wish to donate an organ. These good-hearted people are willing to endure physical pain and personal risk for the sake of doing something to help others.

A prevalent view in the medical community and society in general is that someone who wants to undergo risk and suffering in order to donate a kidney to an unknown recipient must be mentally unbalanced. I regret this cynical perspective. A person who runs into a burning building to save a child is awarded a medal for bravery! To me, it is perfectly understandable that an altruistic individual might choose to save another's life by means of the rational act of donating an organ. The medical profession should take a long hard look before turning down such offers.

The issue becomes extremely complicated, however, when a price is placed on human organs and a broker is involved. Andrew Schneider, a Pulitzer prizewinner, and his colleague Mary Pat Flaherty clearly document this problem in *The Challenge*

of a Miracle: Selling the Gift (the Pittsburgh Press, 1985). This series
of newspaper articles describe abuses of living donation throughout the world, for example, the buying and selling of kidneys. In
India, lists of potential donors from whom kidneys can be pur-
chased, have been published, detailing the donors' names, addresses and tissue types. In India and Pakistan, advertisements
appear regularly in publications, offering kidney donors $1,000
to $7,000 (U.S.). In these countries, an organ broker invariably
arranges for the donor to go to a hospital in India or England,
and, of course, the broker collects a good portion of the payment.

Until recently, some of these operations were done in a legitimate transplant unit, but a ruse was required. The individual
selling the kidney was portrayed as a relative of the recipient, and
falsified documents supported this claim.

At first consideration the practice of selling organs appears
repugnant and unacceptable. However, another viewpoint has
been adopted by responsible members of the Indian medical
community. Picture a poverty-stricken, 18-member extended
family living in India, in which the only breadwinner, the father,
is barely able to eke out a living. If the father decided to take a
job in the mines, a job that involves a risk of death (exceeding
the risk that he would encounter if he donated an organ), we
would laud him for his selfless commitment to his family. If, on
the other hand, he responded to a newspaper advertisement
offering him up to $7,000 (U.S.) — a sum that would give him
lifelong financial security — the western world would judge
him harshly.

I believe that we cannot impose our cultural values on individuals from a different society. And before some of us become
self-righteous in our reaction to the monetary gain realized by
the selling of organs in India, we must remember that most
medical caregivers throughout the world profit from services
rendered. That, at least in North America, is one by-product of
the health care industry. The reality is that doctors usually profit

from patients' illnesses and, of course, corporations profit from the manufacture of drugs and other health care products, which in turn are sold by brokers and wholesalers, while landlords and developers profit from the selling of space for hospitals, all part of the business of providing care to the sick.

Nonetheless, a major problem in the buying and selling of organs is that the recipient remains wealthy on all counts while the destitute seller ultimately loses that which cannot be replaced: a kidney. Also, if a buyer pays $7,000 (U.S.) for a kidney, the donor often receives no more than $2,000. And the medical care that the seller receives is frequently inadequate. If this practice is to be condoned in societies that deem it to make sense, then it should more adequately acknowledge the true risk and worth of the transplant process, and the seller should receive the best medical care possible. These societies should work out a morally justifiable method for potential recipients to pay into the system, while at the same time ensuring the highest level of medical care and adequate compensation for the seller. For example, if wealthy recipients wish to purchase donor organs, they might be required to pay into the system not only enough money for their own organ transplant but also enough to pay for a poor person's transplant as well.

To me, the most questionable aspect of this buying and selling is that a middleman or a broker makes money by trading in human flesh. Schneider and Flaherty's most shocking example of the abusive commercialization of organ-trading involved a broker in Japan. A loan shark, this broker had set up computerized lists of individuals who owed money to other loan sharks. Each debtor had been tissue-typed and assigned a dollar value on the basis of health, age, tissue match and, most importantly, how much the debtor owed the loan shark. There was absolutely no concern whether the donor was at all suitable, so that a potential recipient risked getting a kidney that was less than ideal. The most offensive aspect of this form of commercialization is that the primary goal of medical care should be alleviating human suffering, not increasing it.

GUIDELINES FOR DONATIONS

Society in general and the medical community in particular have been unprepared to deal with the complexities arising from the fast pace of organ transplant research breakthroughs. To help governments, courts, doctors, hospitals and patients to deal with the question of ethics (what should be done?) as well as the question of process (how should it be done?), a set of guidelines has been established by the Transplantation Society.

These guidelines are intended to standardize the ethics of organ donation and to curb potential abuse throughout the world. They have been published and adopted generally by medical communities in the western world. They include both guidelines for distribution of cadaveric organs and guidelines for donation of kidneys by unrelated living donors.

While the Society has no legal authority to insist that a country adopt its recommendations, it can exert peer pressure upon its members to uphold them. If a member does not maintain the Society's published standards, the Society can expel that doctor or physician and announce the expulsion to its members.

Following are the Transplantation Society's guidelines for organ distribution:

1. *The best possible use must be made of the donor gift.*
2. *Organs should be transplanted to the most appropriate recipient on the basis of medical and immunological criteria.*
3. *Useable organs should never be wasted. In the majority of cases, an organ will be used within an established regional or national organ sharing network, and only if it cannot be placed should it be offered to other credible networks, and then only to non-profit centres.*
4. *Sharing of organs should only be arranged via national and/or regional organ sharing networks.*
5. *Priorities in the assignment of organs cannot be influenced by political considerations, gifts, special payments or by favoritism to special groups.*

6. *Transplant surgeons/physicians should not advertise regionally, nationally or internationally.*

The Transplantation Society's guidelines for donation of kidneys by unrelated living donors are as follows:

1. *Living unrelated donors (i.e., not first degree relatives) should be used exceptionally when a satisfactory cadaver or living related donor cannot be found.*
2. *It must be established by the patient and transplant team alike that the motives of the donor are altruistic and in the best interest of the recipient and not self-serving or for profit. In the best interests of all concerned, the motivation and medical suitability of the donor should be evaluated by physicians independently of the potential recipient, the recipient's physicians and the transplant team. An independent donor advocate should be assigned to the unrelated donor to ensure that informed consent is made without pressure, to enhance personal attention given to the donor through the entire donation period, to ensure official expressions of gratitude and to aid with subsequent problems or difficulties. In all instances, and especially in the exceptional case where the emotionally related donor is not a spouse or second degree relative, the donor advocate would ensure and document that the donation was one of true altruism and not self-serving or for profit.*
3. *Active solicitation of living unrelated donors for profit is unacceptable.*
4. *Living unrelated donors must be of legal age.*
5. *The living unrelated donor must satisfy the same ethical, medical and psychiatric criteria used in the selection of living related donors.*
6. *It should be clearly understood that no payment to the donor by the recipient can be allowed. However, reimbursement for*

loss of work earnings and any other expenses related to the donation is acceptable.

7. *The diagnostic and operative procedures on the donor and recipient must be performed only in recognized institutions whose staff are experienced in living related donations and transplantation. It would be expected that the donor advocate should be a member of the same institution but not a member of the transplant team.*

Special Resolution

No transplant surgeon/team shall be involved directly or indirectly in the buying or selling of organs/tissues or in any transplant activity aimed at commercial gain to himself/herself or an associated hospital or institute. Violation of these guidelines by any member of the Transplantation Society may be cause for expulsion from the Society.

We grapple constantly with the problem of those who wish to donate a kidney to a loved one but whose tissue may not match. Dr. Felix Rapaport, past president of the Transplantation Society and a highly regarded international transplant surgeon, has proposed a unique way to assist these individuals, by enabling them to donate one of their kidneys to an international pool.

The system would work like this: Suppose an individual has a loved one — either a spouse or family member — on dialysis, and for some medical reason that loved one is unable to accept the relative's donor kidney. The relative could register with an international computerized kidney bank, indicating willingness to donate a kidney. He or she would be checked to ensure medical fitness. The person's tissue type and blood group would be entered into the kidney bank's files.

Somewhere else in the world, another relative in a similar predicament would also have registered with the international kidney bank. A careful cross-check would verify that the best possible match between donor and recipient was made. The identities of the two donors and recipients would never be revealed, but the two loved ones would be saved by receiving a medically compatible kidney.

The two donors would go into an operating theater at the same time and each would have a kidney removed. Each kidney would be perfused, placed in a container and flown to the city where the recipient lived. The two recipients would then go into operating rooms to receive a kidney transplant. In spirit, they would have received the kidney of their relative. In reality, they would have received a kidney from an unknown but generous donor.

This creative solution would be expensive, but not much more costly than current methods of transporting kidneys. Based on goodwill and charity, this method would provide the benefit of the best possible organ match.

If organ donation does not increase in the way in which I believe it can and should, then this type of proposal should be carefully considered.

BRAIN DEATH

THROUGHOUT RECORDED HISTORY, and until recent years, breathing was considered the definitive sign of life. A pronouncement of death was based on placing shiny objects beneath the nostril and observing that no breath clouded the shiny surface. When William Harvey discovered the circulatory system in 1627, the heartbeat was recognized as another vital sign, and the absence of these two responses — breathing and heartbeat — became the operative definition of death.

With the advent of respirators, cardiac resuscitation and pacemakers in the 1960s, the criteria for pronouncing death had to change because the heart could now be made to function through artificial means. The medical community needed a new definition. Hence, the concept of brain death: the irreversible cessation of brain function that is equivalent to death even though the heart may continue to beat because of a respirator.

The brain death criterion goes beyond examining the heart and lungs to determine that they have stopped. It calls for testing to assure the doctor that all tests of brain function are negative, and irreversibly so. Whether or not other body organs — including heart and ventilator-assisted lungs — are functioning, the patient has definitely died at some point and is now unquestionably and irrevocably dead.

It is important to note that in all of this the doctor is not saying *when* the patient died, but simply verifying that at the time of examination the patient is *now* dead. Death, by this definition, is recognized for what it is: a process, not an event such as cessation of heartbeat. We have come to realize that the creeping process of death reaches a point at which two criteria are met: the whole brain is dead and the process is irreversible.

The modern era of "whole brain death" diagnosis has made vital organ transplantation possible. Indeed, in societies such as Japan, where until recently brain death was not accepted as a means of defining death, only kidney and cornea transplants could be performed, because by the time the heart had stopped and the diagnosis of death had been made, all other vital organs were irretrievably damaged.

The brain's function can be largely divided into two categories: the vegetative or integrating functions; and the conscious or cognitive functions. It is important to note the differences in the two functions. For example, the vegetative functions control breathing while the conscious functions control thinking.

Vegetative functions are controlled primarily by the brain stem, a part of the "lower" or "early development" brain at the base of the skull. It can be thought of as the keyboard of a computer. Consciousness and cognitive functions are controlled by the hemispheres of the brain, which can be thought of as the computer itself. Both the "keyboard" and the "computer" are needed in the integrated, sustained recognition and thought that comprise human behavior. Unfortunately, the part of the brain that controls the conscious and cognitive functions is sometimes destroyed, while the part of the brain that controls the vegetative functions continues to maintain a body's breathing, temperature and blood pressure.

With the criterion of whole brain death has come a flurry of debate. On one side is the concern that we preserve our understanding of death and protect the precision of diagnosing death by using the whole brain death standard. The other side urges continued exploration of the separation of the vegetative and cognitive functions, and a definition of brain death as the permanent loss of consciousness and cognition. I support the side that says death is death of the whole brain including vegetative and cognitive functions.

DIAGNOSING BRAIN DEATH

Diagnosing brain death must be carefully managed. What seems apparent at first may in fact not be so. A case at our hospital is a prime example of why we follow the procedures of determining brain death very carefully.

An 18-year-old man had been involved in a car accident in a small town outside London, Ontario. He was rushed to hospital, where he lay in a coma. He was put on a respirator and fed intravenous fluids. The coma deepened. The physician discussed the possibility of organ donation with the young man's relatives, and our center was contacted.

In these cases, medical protocol requires that the patient be referred and admitted to hospital under the neurosciences department. Here the patient's condition is diagnosed and decisions are made as to whether or not anything can be done. The neurosurgeons decided to admit the boy to the ICU. Our department received no more calls.

A few days later, I was in the ICU. I noted a healthy 18-year-old sitting on the side of his bed, waiting to be transferred to a room. The nurse informed me that the young man had arrived in a coma and had been considered a possible organ donor. Quite properly, I had never been informed of the young man's arrival at the hospital, nor of his progress. It was none of my business.

The story then unfolded. Upon admission the young man was in a deep coma and was placed on a respirator. When the ICU doctor and the neurosurgeon examined him, they declared him to be in a deep coma, but not brain-dead. They did not know the cause of coma. When the patient was tested, he still had brain stem reflexes and the EEG proved positive. But blood tests revealed his sodium (salt) levels were extremely high, which accounted for his deepening coma state. The high sodium content in his IV fluids only served to worsen his condition.

When the IV fluids were changed, the patient woke up in two days and was back home in a week. In fact, his original head injury was not of great significance, apart from contributing to his unconscious state.

The current criteria used in diagnosing brain death are extremely rigorous and conservative. The assumption that the whole brain, both the vegetative and cognitive parts, must be totally destroyed to constitute death goes beyond what some people would consider necessary. The main point, however, is that no mistake can be made. If strict criteria are met, families will be more likely to donate the organs of relatives declared brain-dead in order to save the lives of others.

The Harvard Ad Hoc Committee on Brain Death developed criteria of brain death to reassure the public that strict guidelines are being followed. The guidelines insure that the diagnosis is made by two physicians who are independent of the transplant team. The public can be assured that in reputable medical centers where transplants are carried out, no life will be endangered by a hasty or mistaken diagnosis, or worse, one that is biased.

We do occasionally hear stories in which people are pronounced dead and later come to life in a morgue or hospital. These involve cases in which the original diagnosis was not that of brain death but was based on a state of coma that later reversed itself, or a situation in which the arrested heart reversed itself. Neither of these situations, to my knowledge, would have passed a properly conducted brain death examination.

Some spinal cord reflexes may continue after the patient is thought to be dead. The limbs can be drawn up due to a muscle spasm and a long exhalation of breath can rattle in the throat. Also, in observing a person in deep coma caused by poisoning or drowning, a physician can initially be fooled, on the basis of a cursory examination, into believing that brain stem death has occurred. These situations require prolonged observation in order to confirm, once the effects of poisoning or drowning have passed, that the whole brain is truly dead.

Various tests of brain stem function can be carried out at the bedside, such as examining the nerve connecting the inner ear and the eyes. This is done by putting ice-cold water into the ear canal and watching for movement of the eyes to that side. (No movement indicates a lack of functioning in the brain stem.) This test, along with an EEG (brain tracing) and cessation of breathing when the patient is taken off the respirator, provides absolute proof to the doctor that brain death has indeed occurred.

In summary, the following criteria must be satisfied for the diagnosis of brain death:

- A cause of brain death has been established but patients with potentially reversible conditions (such as hypothermia and drug intoxication) are not to be declared brain dead.
- The patient has no response to painful stimuli and no spontaneous movements.
- Brain stem reflexes are absent (i.e., pupils are unreactive to light and there is no eye movement in response to tests, as in the above example).
- The patient is apneic (not breathing) when taken off the respirator under conditions that meet the official guidelines.
- These criteria must persist when the patient is evaluated again at a later time.
- If the patient is to be considered as a potential organ donor, two physicians unrelated to the transplant team must make their separate diagnoses.

Sometimes, special tests are used, such as the electroencephalograph, which records brain waves, and cerebral angiography or radionuclide scintigraphy, both of which indicate absence of blood flow in the brain.

A proper and complete diagnosis of brain death is a sure safeguard that no life will be terminated that could have been saved. The attending physician should assure the family of a potential donor that all the criteria have been met and that details are readily available if they should require even more reassurance.

THE PVS DILEMMA

The application of the whole brain death concept is a workable model and addresses the needs and safety of all. However, there are two unusual types of patients we hear a great deal about: those in a persistent vegetative state (PVS) and the anencephalic — babies born without a whole brain. Both types of patients address the question of upper brain death, that affecting the cognitive and consciousness functions.

Some people in the medical field suggest discarding the idea of whole brain death and replacing it with a view that death is a permanent loss of consciousness and cognition. However, most members of the medical community agree that for the time being and for the foreseeable future, brain stem death should be a prerequisite for confirming the diagnosis of brain death.

Those patients who have sustained an irreversible brain injury in which their cognitive abilities have been destroyed, but in which their brain stem continues to function, are in what is called the persistent vegetative state, or PVS. There are about 10,000 PVS patients in the United States and Canada who remain permanently unconscious in nursing homes and chronic care hospitals, in some cases up to 30 years. The cost of this to relatives and to society is enormous. These patients lie, mindless, in back wards of institutions, fed by unseen, unfelt hands and cleaned of body wastes by workers they will never know. But as vegetative organisms they continue to live. To extinguish their lives would be homicide.

At the 1989 congress on Ethics, Justice and Commerce in Transplantation, held in Ottawa, the consensus was that these patients were *not* potential donors of organs, because medical science does not know with absolute certainty when the diagnosis can be made that no future cognitive activity in these patients could ever occur. If this certainty existed, then the acceptance of PVS as a form of death might be more thinkable. But no room for error can be allowed. Certainly, considering PVS patients as irrevocably dead is not to be encouraged by the transplant community, despite the obvious benefits to be derived from such a change in thinking.

ANENCEPHALY

There is a condition at birth that has some similarities to the persistent vegetative state. It has been a subject of controversy with regard to transplantation, both for medical scientists and the public. This is the condition known as anencephaly, which occurs in a baby born without a whole brain.

This tragedy occurs in three of every 10,000 births in North America, with about one-third of these babies alive at birth. For unknown reasons, both the higher brain and the skull fail to form; this abnormality occurs as early as at 16 to 22 days of gestation.

Anencephaly is a condition that can be diagnosed with certainty before birth by an ultrasound and blood test. If the condition is diagnosed before birth, an increasing number of women choose to abort. Those infants who are born, although lacking a skull and the hemispheres of the brain, spontaneously move their limbs, suck, respond to sounds (an evidence of a reflex), and breathe spontaneously. This is because the reflex centers responsible for breathing and sucking are located in the brain stem. As long as the brain stem functions, the signs of vegetative life will remain. But the baby will usually die within days.

Some authors, including Michael Harrison of the University of California, San Francisco, Robert Truog of Harvard and John Fletcher of the University of Virginia, suggest that because an anencephalic does not possess a brain, the essence of life can never be realized. They suggest that anencephalics "lack temporal functional integrity" and, therefore, like brain-dead patients, they should be placed in a special category of brain death because they will never achieve cognitive function.

In an attempt to fulfill the wishes of mothers who want something good to come out of their pregnancy after they learn their child will be born without a brain, the University Hospital in London, Ontario and Loma Linda University Medical Center in California initiated a plan at least partially to alleviate the grief of those with anencephalic babies. In January, 1987, a group of scientists, physicians and philosophers met at the University Hospital to consider whether the usual criteria of brain death, that is, total brain death including the brain stem, could be used in an experimental protocol that respected the rights of anencephalic babies, was sensitive to the needs of the mother and was technically possible. Guidelines were established both in Loma Linda and in London to provide for a clinical protocol.* Of the first 12 anencephalics born in the Loma Linda hospital, only two were potential donors; but of the first four anencephalics born in London, using the agreed-upon clinical protocol, two became donors.

The first offer to donate organs from a baby without a brain came from Fred and Karen Schouten of Barrie, a small town in Ontario. The couple had gone to their family doctor because the baby didn't seem to be moving normally. An ultrasound showed that the baby had no brain. When the couple were told that the baby they had longed for would not live, Fred and Karen asked the doctor if the organs of their baby could be used to give life to another baby.

The baby girl was born as predicted, an anencephalic. But for that couple, she was nevertheless their baby. They tenderly picked up the little one, cradled her and loved her. They carried her over to the window and named her Gabriel, after the guardian angel.

Our unit received a call from the obstetrician and the family doctor. They explained that an anencephalic baby had been born and that following a period of shock, the baby had recovered and was breathing. Was it possible, they asked, that the organs could be used? I explained the criteria that we had

*   Stiller, C.R., T. Frewen, T.O. Marshall. *Transplantation Proceedings* 1988; 20 (4 Supplement 5): 79-80.

established, just months earlier, in order to deal with the anencephalic as a donor. My colleague, Dr. Tim Frewen, arranged for the baby to be brought under his care at the pediatric care unit of the Children's Hospital of Western Ontario. On the third day Gabriel stopped breathing. An independent neurologist examined her and declared her brain-dead.

I called Dr. Leonard Bailey in Loma Linda, California and told him that we had a potential donor. At the hospital there a woman from Vancouver was near term with a baby whose heart chambers had not formed, yet who seemed perfectly formed in every other way. This condition is fatal to the newborn, in most cases, within hours or days. The statistical chances that a donor would become available in time to save this baby were remote. Therefore, Dr. Bailey agreed to accept Gabriel as a potential donor. She was flown from London, Ontario to Loma Linda.

We anxiously awaited the report from the team I had sent down to accompany Gabriel. At Loma Linda, Gabriel was re-examined and the diagnosis of brain death was confirmed.

When baby Paul was born by Cesarean section, his chest was immediately opened. Gabriel's perfect heart, capable of sustaining life for many years, was taken from her and placed in the baby boy's tiny chest.

The transplant was successful. Baby Paul was soon discharged from hospital and sent home to Canada. Tragically, six weeks later Fred died of a heart attack. But Fred and Karen had shared the joy of knowing that their baby Gabriel had given life to another.

The night Gabriel's parents received the call saying that brain death had been pronounced and that baby Gabriel was on her way to Loma Linda to donate her heart to baby Paul, Fred and Karen had celebrated their baby and her extraordinary life. As Fred so eloquently had put it, "Many of us live a lifetime trying to do something profound. Baby Gabriel, in her two short days, contributed more than many of us will all our lives."

The Fetus And
Other Species
As Donors

SOME TIME AGO A WOMAN asked if her daughter, a young diabetic teenager, could potentially receive islet transplants from fetal tissue as a form of treatment. Islets are the small islands of tissue that produce insulin in the pancreas. Sections of the pancreas are taken from the fetus and placed in a petri dish and cultured from one to two weeks to reduce the chance of rejection. They are then transplanted into the pancreas of a diabetic. Eventually these islets will partially or completely relieve the diabetic from having to take insulin injections.

The answer to the mother's question was "yes." If satisfactory fetal tissue could be found, then the transplant could be done. The mother offered a solution, logical to some, yet troublesome in its conclusions. She proposed that she would become pregnant by her husband, who was also the father of her daughter. If the tissue type of the fetus was identical to her teenage daughter's, she would arrange for abortion just prior to 20 weeks. The pancreas from her fetus would then be transplanted to her daughter. And because the tissues of both the donor (the aborted fetus) and the recipient (the teenage daughter) would be identical, no rejection would occur. Research indicated that this proposal could be carried out, but the ethics in such a case are controversial at best.

Given the severe shortage of donor organs, transplant specialists are compelled to look for other sources. Fetal cells are very attractive for scientific research and therapy because once these cells are placed in an adult body they grow very quickly and become mature, functioning units. Because of its enormous potential for growth, unused fetal tissue is an obvious source of transplantable tissue.

Most transplants from a fetus are tissues, not organs. One tissue frequently transplanted are islets from the pancreas. If transplantation of islets were permitted, more than 1 million people would benefit from this transplant procedure in North America alone. That number increases by 50,000 per year.

Other transplant possibilities using fetal cells include thymus and liver cells to treat leukemia, aplastic anemia and thalassemia. As long ago as 1958, a patient in Boston received a fetal liver and spleen transfusion in an attempt to treat leukemia. Researchers are also investigating the use of fetal brain cells to treat Parkinson's disease and Alzheimer's disease. One of the most potentially beneficial fetal transplants is the repair of stroke or spinal cord injuries, in an effort to restore mobility to paraplegics.

THE FETUS AS DONOR

The idea of transplanting tissue from aborted fetuses evokes a number of contradictory responses. Scientists are interested in using discarded tissue to inhibit the progress of debilitating diseases and to cure several death-inducing diseases. Governments could potentially view fetal-cell transplants as a means of reducing medical costs for long-term patients. And those who support unrestricted access to abortion see these transplants as a positive outcome of the painful decision to have an abortion.

However, for people disturbed by the possible linkage of abortion clinics to transplant units and, thus, the procurement

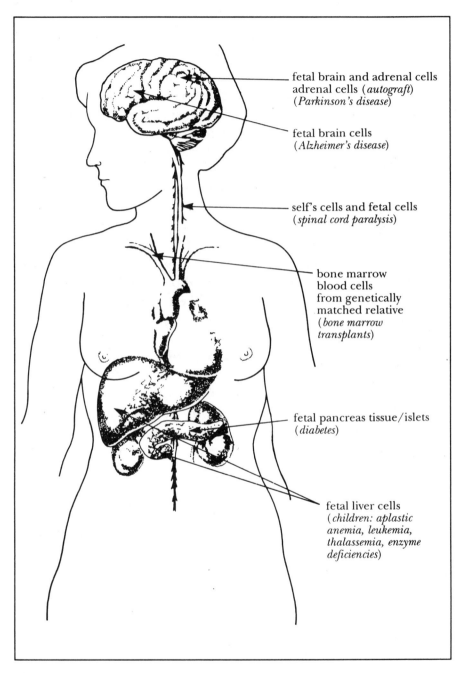

fetal brain and adrenal cells
adrenal cells (*autograft*)
(*Parkinson's disease*)

fetal brain cells
(*Alzheimer's disease*)

self's cells and fetal cells
(*spinal cord paralysis*)

bone marrow
blood cells
from genetically
matched relative
(*bone marrow
transplants*)

fetal pancreas tissue/islets
(*diabetes*)

fetal liver cells
(*children: aplastic
anemia, leukemia,
thalassemia, enzyme
deficiencies*)

Overview of cell transplantation.

of fetal life, this subject is contentious. Since the medical community is committed to protect, enhance and preserve life, some opponents do not tolerate the "using" of one life to preserve another in this way. Respect for the unborn is key to understanding the tension between the benefits of using fetal tissue and the dangers of permitting such procedures. The rights of the unborn are at the center of all ethical and moral concerns about using the fetus as donor.

How are we to make sense of the conflicting views surrounding the use of a fetus? We do know that from conception to birth, the fetus has the potential of developing into a living human being with complete body functions. This is the crux of the difficulty for medical science in the potential use of fetal tissue for therapy and research. In its essential biological makeup, the fetus is human. Its growing physical likeness to a newborn is a constant reminder of its human nature.

There are three basic views in relation to the rights of a human fetus. First, a fetus from the moment of conception has the inherent right to live and should not be interfered with by mother or physician, unless the mother's life is at serious risk.

The second view argues that while the fetus has the inherent qualities of a fully developed individual, it should nevertheless be viewed as a *potential* individual only, and accorded rights at some point in its gestation. That "point," however, is disputed. Some physicians identify brain development — around eight weeks — as the beginning of the individual's existence. They argue that if we regard complete brain death as the end of life, we should therefore regard the beginning of brain activity as the beginning of life.

The third view is that the fetus is human in a cellular sense, but because it is only a collection of cells it has no inherent value until birth.

These viewpoints will continue to be debated as governments and courts make often contradictory decisions, upon which both the medical community and the public must make their own choices.

FETAL TISSUE TRANSPLANTS AND ABORTION

It is important that we distinguish the various reasons that abortions occur. First, there is the spontaneous abortion, and, second, the therapeutic abortion performed to save the life of the mother. In these two situations, the aborted fetus is viewed as a dead person. Thus the use of tissue, if approved of by the mother, elicits little negative public reaction. There is no essential difference between a dead fetus (resulting from an abortion performed to save the life of the mother) and a brain-dead adult who has either consented to donate before death or for whom consent has been given by relatives. In saving the life of the mother, there is almost universal agreement that if a choice has to be made concerning which life should be saved, the mother takes priority. These two situations, however, account for less than one percent of all abortions.

The really problematic situation, and the one that accounts for almost all abortions, is elective abortion. In North America there are more than one and a half million abortions per year. Given the enormous possibilities both for therapy and research, the question being advanced by many organizations is, why not derive some benefit from these abortions? They ask that those with incurable diseases be allowed access to the tissues of hundreds of thousands of fetuses that otherwise are simply discarded.

This leads to another problem. Because the tissue must be in good condition for successful transplantation, the abortion method must not lacerate the fetus. Current methods do not often produce fetal tissue that is useable in transplants. Refinements in the process of inducing an abortion will be necessary if widespread usage of fetal tissue is to be successful.

The third form of abortion is what is called the "designer abortion," in which a fetus is developed for the specific purpose of providing tissue for a specific person. The woman who wanted to get pregnant in order to use fetal tissue to cure her diabetic daughter was proposing such an abortion.

One argument maintains that such a process is not only legitimate but desirable: if elected abortion is permitted in the social, psychological or economic interests of the mother, doesn't it therefore make sense to allow the production of a fetus with the express purpose of saving a dying patient from an incurable disease? Add to that the possibility that the person in need of transplant therapy might be a mother or father with dependent children.

The National Institutes of Health in the United States asked a group of distinguished medical, scientific, legal and religious leaders to prepare a report on the use of fetal tissue for transplantation. The result was a two-volume report called *Report of the Human Fetal Tissue Transplantation Research Panel,* December, 1988, published in Bethesda, Maryland. This study describes two opposing sides: those who favor government research funding for fetal tissue transplants and those who oppose government support. The two opposing viewpoints are instructive in shaping our own personal views, as well as medical, legal and political policies.

• *Use of fetal tissue from elective abortions should be permitted for the following reasons:*
1. There is so much potential good that can result from allowing fetal tissue to be transplanted. While we acknowledge the stress that abortion creates for the mother and others, there exists an opportunity for greater good to be brought to millions of people.
2. The results of this practice can potentially cure diseases and save lives. Therefore we should pursue its advancement. To say no would be to impede the advance of science.
3. Currently, in most countries, it is legal to have an abortion. Thus, an aborted fetus should be regarded as brain-dead and treated in the same way as a cadaveric donor.
4. In western countries there is no dominant religion or ideology to define morality. In a secular environment, the courts of law define and uphold beliefs. If the law does not define

abortion as a criminal act, then abortion is not to be regarded as immoral. Thus, using tissue from an elective abortion should not be considered unethical.

5.   There is no common agreement as to when a fetus, in the course of its gestational development, is determined to be a person. This lack of consensus puts the burden of proof for not using fetal tissue on the shoulders of those who oppose it. Given the lack of consensus, it is logical to allow science to carefully experiment with and use fetal tissue for therapy.

• *Use of fetal tissue from elective abortions should not be permitted for the following reasons:*

1.   Given that society cannot agree when life begins, medical science should err on the conservative side in its estimation of the beginning of human life, opting for an earlier rather than a later beginning. It is the mandate of medical caregivers to defend and support the most vulnerable and weakest of humans.

2.   Linking government-sponsored medical programs with the use of fetal tissue derived from elective abortions implies public acceptance of abortion. When prestigious organizations, foundations, legal bodies, medical enterprises and government task forces unite, this collaboration implies a tacit approval. The widespread use of fetal tissue, especially when approved and funded by the government, would imply the acceptance of abortion as legitimate.

3.   There is a very real concern that if abortion clinics and transplant units are connected through obtaining and using fetal tissue, a dependency between the two will be established. This linkage will, it is feared, engender a medical industry of transplantation that can continue only if abortion clinics continue to supply tissue.

4.   If aborted fetal tissue is used for therapy or research, it will ease the mother's mind, who by believing that ultimate benefit is being realized from her elected abortion will therefore find justification for the abortion.

5. Because society has been unable to reach a consensus as to when the developing unborn child is fully human, medical science should go out of its way to ensure that there is no violation of the unborn even if the objective is to bring a cure to others.

6. The arguments supporting use of fetal tissue are based on a pragmatic, materialistic and utilitarian view — it's available, it's legal, it works — that regards life as being purely physical. This viewpoint fails to recognize the spiritual component of life.

The issues of abortion and the use of fetal tissue are not mutually exclusive. As a doctor and scientist involved in organ transplantation, I cannot pretend that the moral concerns I have regarding abortion are separate from the use of fetal tissue resulting from elective abortion. We are torn between providing therapy to save people who may die unless a transplant is received, and resisting the pressure of organizations and interest groups who want unrestricted use of fetal tissue for purposes of research and therapy.

It is important that the institutions that perform abortions and those that perform fetal tissue transplants be kept completely separate. There are too many possibilities for financial gain if abortion facilities are linked to transplant units. Thus, if there is any utilization of fetal tissue for therapy or research, a neutral mediating agency such as the Red Cross must guard against potential commercialization and abuse.

We must ensure that human values and societal practices are not shaped primarily by the scientific community. The science of organ transplantation, like nuclear science, must be accountable to society. It cannot stand alone, with an open mandate to do what it wants as long as there is progress. Progress defined exclusively as the improvement of technical skills may not be progress at all.

Many people whose intellectual competence and moral

concerns I respect have challenged the use of fetal tissue. We ignore their concerns at our own peril.

It is all too easy to slide the slippery slope of medical ethics. Without clearly defining the source of organs and determining that they have not come from pregnancies procured for donation, we will destroy our ethical credibility. Even though we know the potential benefits to those afflicted by terrible disorders, these benefits do not automatically legitimize the use of tissue from the unborn.

As in the sale of kidneys, when someone wants an organ and is prepared to pay the price, someone else will be willing to sell. And the potential profit from the selling of fetal tissue will escalate as people recognize this as a viable cure. If an unrestricted market in fetal tissue were to spring up, the fetus could become a veritable gold mine for transplantable tissue.

When abortions occur, there should be no opportunity for people to profit financially. In certain permissible circumstances tissue should not be wasted or discarded but used for human benefit. Permission to do this should not rest solely with the mother. In the case of elective abortion, it should be decided by disinterested parties unrelated to either the mother or the transplantation, who can monitor the process and prevent the sale of tissue.

In North America, one and a half million fetuses are aborted each year and treated essentially as tissue for discarding. On the surface, this seems to be an enormous waste of tissue that could be used to cure human disease. Yet there is the frightening danger of wholesale manipulation of the unborn. These complex issues will take years, if ever, to be settled.

USING OTHER SPECIES AS DONORS

The world was shocked when Dr. Leonard Bailey of Loma Linda Hospital in California announced that, having failed to find an appropriate human heart, he had transplanted the heart of a baboon into the chest of newborn baby Fae. He had searched for a human heart of the right size, but none was available. While criticism rained down upon him, his team battled day after day to keep the baboon heart beating in the little girl's chest. Some scientists called the transplant irrational. They reasoned that the possibility of crossing the species barrier was so remote that it was foolish to even try. Animal rights advocates denounced him for sacrificing the heart of an animal for the uncertain future of a human being. Finally baby Fae died of complications with therapy. But we have not heard the last of interspecies transplants. Indeed, one human adult survived 14 months with a baboon heart transplanted by Dr. Mark Hardy and Dr. Keith Reetsma in 1979, again at Loma Linda Hospital.

Interspecies transplants are very complex. Controlling the rejection reaction is extremely difficult. What is particularly interesting in the baby Fae case is that transplanting tissue into a newborn suggests the possibility that the immune system is not yet fully developed at birth. If the baby is young enough, the immune system might accept this type of foreign tissue as self.

Remarkable experimentation is being done on transplanting islets from one species to another. Dr. Kevin Lafferty in Denver has developed a procedure in which islets are taken from mice and put into diabetic rats that are then cured of their diabetes. If this procedure can be extended from an animal to a human, the potential of eliminating diabetes by transplantation may be realized within our lifetime. However, it is one thing to transplant from a mouse to a rat, and another thing to transplant from a rat or a mouse to a human. However, the refinement of this procedure would reduce the demand for fetal tissue transplant, at least in curing diabetes.

The big question is: Should we transplant from one species to another? I believe it is an important question to ask. But when it comes to deciding between the survival of a human or an animal, there is no question in my mind. I choose advancing the life of humans.

The only situation in which interspecies transplants should be considered at present is when human tissue is not available. A nonhuman organ might serve as a bridge until a human organ is found. For example, if a patient urgently requires a heart transplant and no donor is available, the heart of a primate, such as a baboon, may be placed in the patient's chest cavity, taking over the function of the diseased heart until a human heart is found. It *is* conceivable that the science of immunology will advance to the point where nonhuman organs can be transplanted successfully, which would solve much of the current problem of insufficient donor organs.

I believe the difference between human and nonhuman life, or animal life, is that of quality and not quantity, as animal rights activists would want us to believe. When I look through a microscope at the tissue of a human, I recognize that it is from an individual with potential for thought, discerning right from wrong, and establishing moral and spiritual relationships. Although I, too, believe that animals have some rights, it is not a problem for me judiciously to use an animal to support and extend human existence.

For years we have used insulin in humans to control diabetes. Insulin is derived from the pancreas of slaughtered cows and pigs. The "transplanting" of these hormones from animals to humans has never been disputed.

The real issue is the lack of human organs. If people would sign their organ donor cards and if doctors would ask families to donate the organs of their deceased loved ones, the supply of human organs would nullify the question of interspecies transplants.

How Religions
Respond

I T IS A POPULARLY HELD VIEW that organized religions oppose organ donation. In fact, this is not always true. While some religions have no defined view of the body as it relates to organ transplants, most major religions encourage donation.

Here is an example from my own experience of unexpected religious support. I received a call that a potential donor, a victim of a car accident, had been declared brain-dead. I knew that the heart could be used to save the life of a desperately ill young woman at our center. But when the physician from the intensive care unit called, he wasn't optimistic. "Unfortunately, Dr. Stiller," he said, "the potential donor is a Jehovah's Witness." He assumed that a family belonging to this religious group, which believes that the transmitting of human blood or blood products is an offense according to the Bible, would refuse to donate an organ.

A colleague of mine, Dr. Paul Keown, asked a Jehovah's Witness minister to visit the victim's parents and grandparents. Following discussions with the family and consultations with church leaders, the minister made a recommendation that the family should donate. He explained, "We consider it wrong to receive a blood transfusion. But if tissues or organs can be used to help someone else, that is the recipient's problem, not ours."

As a result, the heart of a Jehovah's Witness was transplanted into the body of a Roman Catholic woman.

In outlining the basic views of major religions towards organ transplants, I recognize the danger of making assumptions based on the little I know of their belief structures. I have therefore based the following discussion on material from the *Transplantation Proceedings*, Volume XX, No. 1, Supplement 1, February, 1988, and on the remarks of those who spoke on religious concepts at "Ethics, Justice and Commerce in Transplantation: A Global Issue," a conference held in Ottawa in August, 1989.

JUDAISM

Jewish law, called *Halachah*, affirms that the preservation of life is a priority in Jewish ethics. Of primary concern to Judaism is the preservation and enhancing of life, and second, the preservation of the dignity of a person's physical being. So, for example, an executed criminal is not to be left hanging overnight but must be buried before sundown.

In Judaism, the important religious consideration when a living person donates a kidney is the amount of risk to the donor weighed against the benefit to the recipient. Given the preciousness of human life and the mandate to maintain and enhance it, a donor may take a calculated risk if benefit to the recipient is probable. Therefore, as the risk to donors decreases over time due to advances in medical technology, the equation is tipping in favor of living organ donation.

Central to Jewish concerns about organ donation is whether the donor is dead. Removing organs after death is a potential problem in Judaism, for three reasons: it may be viewed as desecrating the body; there is a prohibition against deriving any benefit from a corpse; and Jewish law prescribes that the deceased be given a full burial. To take organs from a dead body may violate these Jewish norms, according to comments made by Rabbi Dr. Reuver P. Bulka in Ottawa (August, 1989). Jewish law prohibits the encouragement of death in order that organs can be taken to help someone in need of a transplant. Thus, a careful diagnosis of brain death is essential.

Jewish law is not concerned that transplants interfere with the purposes of God because, since life is a gift from God, so is the enhancement of life. Therefore, while the Jewish religion does not object to the idea of organ transplants, the obstacle is to convince Jews of the many benefits, and further, to persuade them that to donate organs is an act of loving kindness. It is also important to explain that brain death is a more satisfactory definition of death than the cessation of heartbeat and breathing.

In my experience with Jewish donors, the influence of rabbis has been both helpful and proactive. Our profound concern for the maintenance and enhancement of human life has had a great effect on rabbinical participation in these situations. Most rabbis are prepared to override the religious restrictions against mutilating the body and delaying burial, in favor of a concern for the life of the potential recipient, who could be saved by the organs of a deceased donor.

I recently had a patient from New York who had been referred to the University Hospital for surgery on an aneurysm. Unfortunately, the aneurysm ruptured before surgery could be performed and brain death occurred. The patient was an orthodox Jew and it was with some reticence that the staff approached the family. They were anxious about mutilation of the body and whether the body would be buried before sundown the following day.

The deceased was a potential multi-organ donor. The necessity to confirm brain death, coordinate the teams and transfer the body to New York before sundown on the following day made the case especially difficult. The rabbi in attendance emphasized to the family the overriding principle of the value of human life. He stressed that although mutilation of the body was a concern, the more important factor was the opportunity to enhance the life of a living individual.

The conflict in the minds of this orthodox Jewish family was

apparent. But the outcome of the discussion of practical considerations as well as the consolation they received from their rabbi
led them to make every effort to meet the letter of the law while
preserving the spirit of their faith. We even managed to have the
body flown back for burial within the required time.

In this instance, as in many others, the respect for religious law
shown by the medical team enhanced the likelihood of organ
donation and helped the family deal with bereavement.

ISLAM

While Islamic countries have traditionally not donated organs,
it is ironic that the prime purchasers of kidneys have been Islamic
patients who have bought kidneys from countries such as India.
In fact, the threat of an influx of rich Arabs from the Middle East
into the United States seeking to buy American organs precipi-
tated a legislated policy that allowed only 10 percent of those on
American waiting lists to be non-landed immigrants. A rule was
established that all American organs must first be offered to
Americans before they can be sent outside the country.

Until recently, organ donations in Islamic countries have been
virtually nonexistent. The donating of body parts is legal in
Islamic law, with certain prerequisites. But the sale of human
parts is illegal.

Only recently have ethical discussions concerning organ donations been held among Muslim scholars. Thus, it is difficult to
ascertain a single, unified religious perspective. In debating the
medical practice of organ transplants, Muslim scholars and ju-
rists are divided. Some strongly oppose it; others understand the
need for it.

Those who support transplantation argue that it is permissible
because it is not forbidden in the 14th-century Koran (the
prophet Muhammad's teaching in the Islamic Code of Ethics).
If an action has good intentions and does not contradict a basic
principle of Islam, then Islam should encourage such trends. In
the opinion of Islamic proponents of transplantation, removing

an organ from a dead body does not demean the dead. Instead, as part of a process of sharing life, it bespeaks respect for the dead. Since everything in Islam belongs to God, it is the responsibility of the human race to take care of everything entrusted to us by God. Thus, using resources in this way is good and the abuse of this resource is considered a sin.

As in Judaism, Islam requires that the dead be buried as soon as possible after death. Mutilation of the body is also prohibited. The belief that human remains should be kept sacred and intact is attributed to the prophet and founder of Islam, Muhammad. Postmortem examination and dissection are permitted only in very rare cases, such as to retrieve something valuable that might have been swallowed.

As in Judaic law, weighing the risk to the donor against the benefit to the recipient is the important consideration.

A qualification arises if the body part might be placed in the body of a non-Muslim. Some Muslims believe that if cremation of the non-Muslim recipient were to occur in the future, the organ should be taken out and buried separately to protect it.

This complex view of the sanctity of the whole, intact being has not led to a consensus that organ donation is permissible. In the foreseeable future, the Islamic world will turn to the non-Islamic community for the majority of their donor organs.

HINDUISM

There is nothing within the writings or traditions of Hinduism that would specifically disallow organ transplants. The Hindu concept of *dharma*, which can be translated "good duty," suggests that doing good for others is an inherently desirable thing.

While the various strands of Hindu mythology do not give any indication that organ donation is either right or wrong, kidneys have been sold in India, usually by the poor. However, this practice does not seem to have anything to do with Hinduism as such, but is more a question of the need to sell something otherwise not available. Any reluctance concerning transplantation among those in Hindu countries seems to arise more from the newness of this medical procedure rather than from religious scruples.

BUDDHISM

Generally, nations in which Buddhism is the dominant religion have not been involved in organ donation. However, Buddhism does not prohibit the giving or receiving of organs.

In the Buddhist religion, nothing exists independently: all of nature is interdependent. Even though something may appear separate, on close examination it can be seen that its existence is dependent upon other existing or preexisting thoughts, conditions and individuals.

According to Buddhism, the human body is a conglomeration of matter and mind with no permanent connection between the two. What appears to be permanent, the body, is a mere illusion. Life is a continual series of many deaths and rebirths that happen so quickly that an appearance of the continuity of life is created. Death then is only temporary, a transition to the next rebirth. In rebirth there is a new mind-body partnership. The consciousness of this new partnership had left the former partnership in search of something better.

Thus, according to the Buddhist perspective there is nothing particularly sacrosanct about the body or any part of it, whether it is dead or alive. And there is no essential difference between the human body and a rock, apart from the body possessing a mind. Neither does it make any difference whether the body is cremated or used for donor organs. When a person's body parts are made available for organ transplants, this is seen as an act of generosity.

A Buddhist's view of organ transplants suggests that to transplant a body part is only a technical concern, like replacing the carburetor in a car. So also, transplanting an animal organ into a human is simply a technical procedure.

However, if a transplanted organ is rejected, this may indicate a mental incompatibility between donor and recipient. If, for example, an organ taken from a donor whose spiritual state was immoral just prior to death is implanted into a recipient whose state prior to receiving the implant is moral, the transplant may not be accepted. In such a case, the transfer of organs may have a psychological as well as a physical impact on the recipient.

In Japan and China, heart and liver donations are rare. However, this is not necessarily the result of a religious viewpoint but rather of the use of different criteria for determining death. In these countries, death is defined not only by brain death but also by the stopping of the heart. Because a "beating heart" donor is required to obtain other vital organs, the only organs usually available in these countries are the kidneys, which can be taken immediately after the heart has stopped.

CHRISTIANITY

With the exception of Christian Science, Christianity has in general reacted positively towards organ donation. Statements from most leading Christian organizations have stated that organ donation is commendable. In fact, some Christian leaders have been important advocates of organ donation.

In Christianity a person is not seen as a soul trapped within the body, but rather as the integration of both the body and the soul. According to the doctrine of the "Incarnation," Christ is God, taking on human flesh; both fully divine and fully human. This doctrine sanctifies the notion of "the flesh" and elevates it to a place of importance.

The Resurrection (return to life) of Jesus Christ, body and soul, is vital to the understanding of organ transplants within the Christian world. The Resurrection represents the uniting of the physical and spiritual reality of Christ in a new way. Christ vindicates the essential goodness of physical reality and manifests the integration of the spiritual with the physical. In Christianity, therefore, the body deserves the highest respect. While the dead body is no longer the person, reverence is still called for in remembrance of the person who was.

The second important theological point is that a future Resurrection has been promised for all. The soul is not complete until it is reunited with the body. Therefore the dead body is accorded ultimate respect.

Most Christian theologians view the giving of organs as an act of love. The organs that are transplanted are not simply pieces of equipment, but part of an eternal person, and therefore, holy.

Of extreme importance is the affirmation that the donor is truly dead. If not, the unity of the body and soul is being violated. The definition of what is meant by brain death is critical to Christian faith. Respect for next of kin is also vital, in that it acknowledges the value and importance of the donated organ.

RELIGION AND MORAL RESPONSIBILITY

Excluding Islam, most major religions regard organ donation as permissible and even noble.

However, it can be very difficult for a family, anguished over the death of a loved one, to ask permission from a religious leader to donate the organs. The problem is compounded if the religious leader has not come to terms with the subject of transplants, or if the religion does not prescribe an answer. Too often religious leaders fail in their responsibility to move beyond giving permission to actually advocating the donation of organs.

It has always seemed paradoxical to me that while ministers, priests or rabbis conduct a funeral or burial, careful that tradition and liturgy are precisely followed, they ignore the fundamental teachings of their religions, which exhort their followers to minister to the needy and to honor the sanctity of life. There are few, if any, religious leaders who actually take active measures to sensitize their followers to the needs of transplant recipients. The act of saving the life of another by donating an organ following death, seems to me the best and most practical demonstration of faith.

There is no major religious obstacle in North America to the donation of organs on the grounds of doctrine or theology. Both the Jewish and Christian communities affirm that their faiths support the idea of giving an organ, after death, so someone can live.

However, two factors inhibit synagogues and churches from encouraging their members to actively support donation. First is the question of brain death. This issue, unless properly explained, can lead to a great deal of anxiety about the possibility of a loved one being misdiagnosed as dead. Since rabbis, priests and ministers are leaders and teachers, it would seem that the most effective means of communication would be for these leaders to give direct and candid information on what is being done in medicine today. Messages and sermons could also be supported by print material, overheads and slides, which transplant associations can provide for educational purposes.

The second factor is the reluctance of some leaders to actively participate in what are thought of as nonreligious activities. I want to advance the notion that to give an organ so someone else can continue to live is by its very nature a religious act. The Rabbi from Nazareth said it well: "No greater love hath a man than this, that he lay down his life for a friend."

ORGAN DONATION IN THE 90S AND BEYOND

SUCCESSFUL KIDNEY TRANSPLANTS began more than 30 years ago and during the 1970s organ transplants became headline news. Initially, transplants were viewed as an experimental and speculative form of treatment, rather than as therapeutic intervention. Therefore, the medical community did not readily accept transplantation as part of their caregiving responsibilities.

It was not until the discovery of the antirejection drug cyclosporine that successful organ transplants became a reality. Organ transplants involving heart, liver and heart and lung began to shed the "experimental" label. Organ transplants became an accepted therapeutic treatment for organ failure and began to contradict the conclusion that the only alternative for those with organ failure was death.

As science has advanced, people have become aware of the great need for organ and tissue supplies. Buoyed by a media interested in the details of donor families and transplant recipients, this increased awareness has pushed the problem of supply into public forums and has forced governments to begin to respond.

Where will we be by the end of the 1990s? Given that vital organs can be transplanted with a success rate of 75 percent, patients should no longer accept noncompliance from their doctors when asked to be referred for an organ transplant.

As well, treatment by transplantation will not be conducted in some faraway medical center, reserved for an elite few. Transplants will occupy the same category as coronary bypass surgery today. And more and more communities will insist on their right to have a transplant facility in their region.

With the increase in public awareness and the corresponding responsiveness on the part of donor families, the donor supply problem will be solved eventually. It is increasingly common for parents to initiate the process by requesting that their infants' organs be retrieved. Of the 25,000 patients who experience kidney failure each year in North America, 20,000 will receive a kidney transplant within the year they are diagnosed. Of the 30,000 patients each year who suffer liver failure, approximately 11,000 should be eligible and will receive a transplanted liver. Of the 550,000 patients who die of heart failure each year, 25,000 to 75,000 will be potential heart candidates and 12,000 will receive a new heart.

For patients with acute liver failure and for children with liver failure, there will be stopgap procedures. Cultured liver cells will be inserted into the abdomens of children with liver disease. These cells will serve as a bridge to supply essential liver function until a new liver is found. Many small children will receive half a liver taken from an adult. And children with enzyme defects will have their deficiency treated by liver cell transplants.

All patients dying of brain death under age 60 will have their hearts examined by sophisticated techniques and, where necessary, repaired, so that their hearts can be donated to someone in need. We will be able to implant an artificial heart, possibly as a longterm solution, but certainly as a stopgap for patients dying of acute coronary thromboses who are waiting for donor hearts. And the 500 to 1,000 neonates born with a life-threatening heart defect will receive heart grafts from cadaveric donors, anencephalic babies and ultimately from animals.

With the increased demand for transplants, where will we find enough donor organs to meet this massive need? Each year in North America there are 30,000 potential kidney donors making up to 60,000 kidneys available. In hospitals where physicians ask relatives for organ donations, 80 percent of the potential organs available can be obtained. This percentage will not be achieved immediately in North America, but by the mid-1990s, we antici-pate that 50 percent of potential donors will offer their kidneys, thus making available some 30,000 kidneys per year.

There are 24,000 potential liver donors each year in North America. With a 50 percent retrieval rate, the lives of 12,000 people per year could be saved.

Diabetics requiring islets to renew their capacity to produce insulin will receive transplants without surgery. By the turn of the century, the supply will be sufficient to treat all diabetics who are on insulin. New cases of insulin-requiring diabetics will dwindle as preventative treatment for diabetes becomes stand-ard. And there will be more corneas available than will be required.

How much will maintaining such a program throughout North America cost? In 1990, the cost of doing a transplant has been reduced since the early days of experimental procedures. This is because many cautionary procedures and protocols were unnecessary and patients were kept in hospital much longer than required. The care of a donor in ICU and organizing the retrieval of an organ are two major components in the cost of transplantation. Today, the total average cost is $36,000 for a kidney, $96,000 for a heart, $91,000 for a liver and $131,000 for a lung transplant. In the U.S., the total annual cost for all transplants is $630 million (U.S.), less than one percent of the total health care expenditures.

Placing a patient on an artificial kidney costs $40,000 per year for the lifetime of the patient. Contrast that with $36,000 — once — for a transplant. The costs of allowing a patient to die of liver or heart failure; keeping a patient alive with oxygen at home

because of lung failure; and dealing with the ravages of diabetes — these costs far exceed the cost of transplantation. There
are few areas in medicine, except for polio vaccination, for
example, where cost-effectiveness and cost-benefit analysis come
out in such favor of new technology, as in organ transplants.

A STRATEGY FOR THE FUTURE

Devising a successful strategy to increase organ and tissue donation calls for an integration of the roles of the voluntary, professional and government sectors. Such a strategy will overcome the
barriers that tend to keep these three sectors apart. The medical
profession needs the community to become enthusiastic about
making organ donation a fact of modern life. The government
can, by means of the public purse, help point the way in encouraging organ transplantation, which will result in a better health
care plan. These sectors need each other and if they coordinate
a common strategy, I believe we will see a transformation of
medical practice by the expanded and efficient use of transplantation.

The obstacles to increased donation are many. While we know
they can be eliminated, this will not happen overnight. Patients
discouraged by the lack of donor organs must understand that
we are in the forefront of a new medical movement and that they
are pioneers. Doctors who wonder why the government doesn't
do more must remember that transplant technology is only three
decades old. Change must be managed with care. Scientific
advances must not get too far ahead of public support or there
could be a backlash in which the public refuses to support organ
donation. Those who want to crash onto the public stage and
press for a more radical response may in fact scare people away
from this crusade for life.

While we are not moving as quickly as I wish, there are signs
that we are finding ways to dispel both public and professional
concerns. Examine the lists of influential public and professional
associations that have endorsed organ donation and transplan-

tation and you'll see that both are becoming better educated and showing remarkable signs of support.

BETTER ENDINGS

As we strive to remove barriers, organ transplants will become a result of good planning and not just luck. Conscious design will eliminate the bad luck from the system and replace it with reasonable hope.

One of my patients, Robert, didn't get his chance at life because of an ineffective system. Robert's parents didn't know about the option of an organ transplant because there was no information center detailing what was available and who required which organ. They were not told how they could gain access to the system in order to be referred to a transplant center. And so, although their son was a perfect candidate for an organ transplant, he died.

Jason and his mother had not been prepared in advance to give. How differently these stories would read if these barriers had been removed.

Let me rewrite the stories of Robert and Jason, assuming that they were living in a world in which a successful organ donor retrieval system had been designed and implemented . . .

After Robert's corrective surgery for congenital heart disease, it was evident that he would not be able to lead a normal life. His parents were called in and told about the option of a heart transplant. They learned that although corrective surgery would prolong their son's life, eventually his heart would fail. The only viable solution was a heart transplant, which would give him an 80 percent chance of living a full life.

After Robert's parents pondered this option, read some material and consulted their doctor, they made an appointment for Robert to be tested at the regional referral transplant center. The cardiologist reviewed the medical and surgical data and then examined Robert. The doctor advised the parents that the corrective surgery already performed on Robert would make a heart transplant more difficult. Despite this minor setback, Robert was a suitable candidate for a heart transplant and the cardiologist recommended that he be placed on the waiting list. Although there would be no immediate attempt to find a donor, Robert would be carefully monitored and as soon as there were signs of heart deterioration, a heart transplant would be pursued.

Robert went back to school. Despite his limited involvement in physical exercise and sports, his parents knew that ultimately he would need more treatment. Soon he showed signs of heart failure; he was coughing at night. The cardiologist noted that the left chamber of the heart was now much larger and fluid was accumulating. He injected medication to make the heart work more efficiently and he removed some of the fluid. A call was put through to the transplant center to report Robert's worsening condition. Robert was now put on the active list in search of a donor.

When Robert and his parents arrived at the transplant center, they were met by the social worker and the recipient coordinator, who took him to the transplant unit. They walked by the exercise room where heart recipients, ranging from age ten to 67, were pedalling exercise bikes, lifting weights and walking a treadmill.

Robert's father stopped to talk to a recipient. His transplant had been an ordeal, but although he had spent three days in the intensive care unit, he was now — only four weeks later — completely well and able to ride an exercise bike!

At the outpatient clinic the family met the transplant surgeon and cardiologist. After reviewing Robert's case, the medical team decided that Robert's condition should not be allowed to deteriorate any further or he would be too ill to undergo surgery. The team agreed that Robert's name should be entered into the central computer list, which was distributed immediately throughout the region and across North America.

The recipient coordinator showed Robert's family the list of patients waiting for a heart. Included on the list were not only Robert's priority rating but also his blood group and body size.

The family left the hospital, well informed and reassured that they would have their turn when a donor heart of the right size and blood group became available.

Robert's parents were given a pocket pager that connected them to the hospital communication network, and the family was advised to live as normally as possible and to wait for the moment when the pocket pager would alert them. At that time they would catch a short flight to the center. In the event that a regular flight could not be obtained, a plane would be sent to pick Robert up in time. They were advised not to leave the country or visit an area where it would be difficult to fly Robert to the center quickly.

The family left the hospital and drove home. They knew they faced a difficult time, but they were relieved that Robert's welfare was being looked after and that he would get a fair chance at finding a donor. They felt in control of the situation . . .

Robert is only half the story. What about Jason? Here is how I would like to rewrite that story . . .

When Jason's mother ran out into the street and held Jason in her arms, she was filled with an icy fear that she was about to lose her only son. She looked at Jason and thought of how precious life was. As she held him, she hoped that a miracle would occur; that his state of unconsciousness would pass and he would come back to her. The ambulance arrived and rushed him to the hospital. From emergency, he was quickly transferred to the intensive care unit. The neurosurgeon examined Jason carefully and scanned the brain to assess the degree of damage. He examined Jason's body and found that disturbing paradox that neurologists see so often: a completely healthy body, but a destroyed brain.

The neurologist and the neurosurgeon recognized the hopelessness of the situation. They discussed the case with the intensive care unit staff and decided to wait until every effort had been made to determine a firm diagnosis of brain death.

The nurse called Dr. George Kennedy and informed him of Jason's condition. He knew that he would most likely find evidence of irreversible brain death. He also knew that his main responsibility was to do everything he could for the patient. But in the event that he was brain dead, he would seek his mother's permission to move the transplant team into place.

Dr. Kennedy arrived at the hospital, examined Jason and confirmed brain death. The nurse indicated that hospital policy in situations in which brain death had occurred or was imminent, was to consult with the physician and the social worker on the organ donor team, to decide what course of action should be taken.

The nurse had reviewed the criteria of potential donors and found that Jason matched them perfectly. Although Jason had had a slight fever on admission, the guidelines indicated this did not preclude him from being considered a donor.

Within minutes, the organ donor team arrived to meet with Dr. Kennedy and the nurse. Kennedy explained that after thoroughly examining the patient, he had confirmed Dr. Keith Sinclair's diagnosis that this patient was brain dead and that there was no chance of recovery.

Dr. Jim Barkin, the physician in charge of the hospital's organ donation consulting team, reviewed the criteria and asked Dr. Kennedy if and when he wished to meet with Jason's relatives. Dr. Kennedy indicated his desire to talk to the mother and give her the chance to gain some consolation from her devastating loss.

A PARADIGM FOR TRANSPLANTATION

The rewritten stories above describe what can happen under the best circumstances. Here is the paradigm we are striving towards: Individuals who wish their organs to be used after death can expect that on suffering a fatal brain injury they will be cared for, but when brain death has occurred, their relatives will be consulted and their organs will be retrieved in a respectful manner, kept in good condition and then distributed to those in greatest need.

From the standpoint of someone who needs an organ transplant, medical treatment will be available. Doctors will attempt to prevent disease in an organ, treat it promptly when it occurs, minimize damage as the disease progresses and replace the organ when necessary. In short, modern medicine will seek to maintain health, not just prevent death.

The future will bring dramatic changes in the process of transplantation. When someone needs an organ transplant, it will not be due to mere chance that in a last-ditch effort they will gain access to a life-restoring organ. We will one day live in a society where organ donation will be the norm, not the exception; a world in which the idea of donating a life-sustaining organ will be as routine as donating a pint of blood; a world in which respect for human life precludes commercial value, the selling of organs or the compromising of ethical and moral values.

I foresee a world in which we replace irreversibly diseased organs in the way we replace a heart valve or a hip today. We will experience a predictable supply of donor organs through a network of retrieval centers. This will allow physicians to care for their patients as transplants become a treatment of choice, carried out before the patient has deteriorated into an invalid.

This predictable supply of available organs will occur because the medical profession and our society abhor the waste of valuable and scarce resources. The same commitment and effort that goes into the saving of a life will be applied to the preservation and retrieval of an organ. The sad refrain, "Every organ wasted is another life lost," will be turned into "Every organ saved is another life given."

Conditions Affecting The Suitability And Maintenance Of An Organ Transplant

Certain conditions may indicate to doctors that a patient is in need of an organ transplant. Listed below are some of these major indicators.

Kidney
- irreversible acute or chronic renal failure (i.e., renal vascular disease, hereditary or toxic nephropathies, trauma or tumor in kidney)

Heart
- end-stage cardiac failure (i.e., cardiomyopathy, coronary artery disease)

Heart-Lung
- any lung disorder which has chronic lung failure with associated cardiac failure (i.e., primary pulmonary hypertension)

Lung
- end-stage lung disease (i.e., cystic fibrosis, pulmonary fibrosis)

Liver
- irreversible acute or chronic liver disease (i.e., primary hepatic malignancy, metabolic disorders, biliary disease)

Pancreas
- type I diabetes mellitus (insulin-dependent)
- end-stage diabetic kidney failure
- threatening progression of complications from diabetes

Eye
- corneal disease (i.e., congenital dystrophies, keratoconus, advanced infections)
- visual handicap

The following are infections and diseases that would disqualify a person from receiving a transplant.

Note: The following are contraindications for all potential recipients:
- active infection
- sepsis (blood-borne infection)
- previous or present malignancy
- current substance abuse
- poor compliance

Heart
absolute
- underlying lung disorder that would prevent a new heart from functioning

relative
- active peptic ulcer
- unresolved pulmonary infarction
- cerebrovascular or peripheral vascular disease
- severe liver or kidney dysfunction

Heart-Lung
- peptic ulcer
- irreversible liver or kidney abnormality

Lung
- any other major system failure (kidney, heart, liver)
- steroid therapy

Liver
- extra-hepatic malignancy
- severe lung or heart disease
- severe kidney impairment (unrelated to liver disease)
- portal vein blockage

Pancreas
- advanced microvascular disease
- coronary artery disease (high risk of perioperative cardiac death)
- advanced pulmonary disease

Eye
- damaged or diseased retina
- total loss of vision from glaucoma
- loss of vision from stroke

Indications that the recipient's body may be rejecting the new organ are:

Kidney
- fever
- chills
- nausea

- fatigue/lack of energy
- increased weight
- pain over kidney
- decreased urine output

Heart
- fever
- irregular or fast heart rate
- progressive weight gain (1 kg/day with ankle swelling)
- shortness of breath with mild exertion
- loss of energy and appetite

Heart-Lung
- fever
- shortness of breath
- loss of appetite

Lung
- fever
- fatigue
- shortness of breath
- aches and pains
- loss of appetite

Liver
- jaundice
- fever
- bloating (weight gain; swollen ankles, hands and/or stomach)
- loss of appetite
- nausea and vomiting
- fatigue (unrelated to activity)

Pancreas
- fever
- abdominal pain and tenderness
- hyperglycemia (high amount of glucose in the blood)

Eye
- redness in eye (that had become white following surgery)
- aching pain in eye
- decreasing visual acuity

Donor Criteria

Criteria	Kidney	Heart	Heart-Lung
Age (has flexible limits)	<70	<60	1-50
Cardiac arrest-resuscitated	Probably OK	Possibly	Possibly
No recent injury/surgery to abdomen	Important	Important	Important
No previous disease of organs	Mandatory	Mandatory	Mandatory
No active infections	Mandatory	Mandatory	Mandatory
No present/history of transmissible diseases	Mandatory	Mandatory	Mandatory
Similar weight/body build	No	Yes	Yes
Compatible blood type	Mandatory	Mandatory	Mandatory
Tests indicating suitability	BP	BP	BP
	Urine output	ECG	ECG
	Urinalysis	Chest x-ray	Chest x-ray
	Serum electrolytes	Arterial blood gases	Chest exam
	Creatinine	echocardiogram	Arterial blood gases
	Urea	coronary	Sputum
	Glucose	angiography	culture

Additional comments:
For the heart and heart-lung:
- No cardiac injections
- No severe, chronic hypertension

Criteria	Lung	Liver	Pancreas
Age (flexible limits)	1-50	<70	<60
Cardiac arrest-resuscitated	Possibly	Probably OK	Probably OK
No recent injury/surgery to abdomen	Extremely important	Extremely important	Important
No previous disease of organs	Mandatory	Mandatory	Mandatory
No active infections	Mandatory	Mandatory	Mandatory
No present/history of transmissible diseases	Mandatory	Mandatory	Mandatory
Similar weight/body build	Yes	Yes	No
blood type compatible	Mandatory	Preferred	Mandatory
Tests indicating suitability	BP ECG Chest x-ray Arterial blood gases Sputum culture	BP Bilirubin AST (SGOT) ALT (SGPT) Alkaline Phosphatase (AP) PT/PTT	BP Serum glucose Serum amylase
Additional comments	No infection	No history of alcoholism	No history of diabetes mellitus

Criteria	Bone	Skin	Eye	Heart Valves
Age of donor	16-70	14-75	No age limit	3 mo.-55
Cardiac arrest	Not applicable: heart-beating cadaver not mandatory			
No recent injury or surgery to abdomen	Not important	Not important	Not important	Not important
No previous disease of organs	Mandatory	Mandatory	Mandatory	Mandatory
No active infections	Mandatory	Mandatory	Mandatory	Mandatory
No present history of transmissible diseases	Mandatory	Mandatory	Mandatory	Mandatory
Similar weight/body build	No	Greater than 100 lbs	No	No
Compatible blood type	No	No	Rarely	No
Additional comments:	No long-term therapy with high-dose steroids No irradiation	No long-term antibiotic therapy No drug abuse No history or present cancer	No chronic central nervous system disease Visual acuity not important	Normal valve function Cardiac arrest does not preclude donation

CANADIAN
TRANSPLANT CENTERS

Province	Hospital	Phone Number	Organ Type
British Columbia	Vancouver General Hospital Heather Pavilion D-10 #19 855 West 12th Ave. Vancouver, B.C. V5Z 1M9	604-875-4111	kidney heart liver heart-lung lung
	The Children's Hospital 4480 Oak St. Vancouver, B.C. V6H 3V4	604-875-2345	kidney (pediatric)
	St. Paul's Hospital 1081 Burrard St. Vancouver, B.C. V6Z 1Y6	604-682-2344	kidney
Alberta	Foothills General Hospital 1403-29th St. NW Calgary, Alta. T2N 2T9	403-270-1110	kidney
	University of Alberta Hospital 112th St. & 83rd Ave. Edmonton, Alta. T6G 2B3	403-432-8822	kidney heart heart-lung liver islet cells
Saskatchewan	University Hospital University Drive Saskatoon, Sask. S7N 0X0	306-244-2323	kidney

Manitoba	Health Sciences Centre 700 William Ave. Winnipeg, Manitoba R3E 0Z3	204-787-3661	kidney
Ontario	Toronto (provincial)	800-387-6673	all organs
	St. Joseph's Hospital 50 Charleton Ave. Hamilton, Ontario L8N 4A6	416-522-4941	kidney
	Kingston General Hospital Stuart St. Kingston, Ontario K7L 2V7	613-548-3232	kidney
	University Hospital Children's Hospital of Western Ontario 339 Windermere Rd. London, Ontario N6A 5A5	519-663-3000	kidney heart heart-lung lung liver bowel
	Ottawa Civic Hospital 1053 Carling Ave. Ottawa, Ontario K1Y 4E9	613-761-4000	kidney
	Ottawa General Hospital 501 Smyth Rd. Ottawa, Ontario K1H 8L6	613-737-7777	kidney (adult and pediatric)
	Ottawa Heart Institute c/o Ottawa Civic Hospital 1053 Carling Ave. Ottawa, Ontario K1Y 4E9	613-761-4629	heart heart-lung
	Toronto Western Hospital 399 Bathurst St. Toronto, Ontario M5T 2S8	416-368-2581	kidney heart
	St. Michael's Hospital 30 Bond St. Toronto, Ontario M5B 1W8	416-364-4000	kidney
	Toronto General Hospital 200 Elizabeth St. Toronto, Ontario M5G 2C4	416-595-3111	kidney lung heart-lung liver

	Hospital for Sick Children 555 University Ave. Toronto, Ontario M5G 1X8	416-597-1500	kidney (pediatric) liver (pediatric)
Quebec	Royal Victoria Hospital 687 Pine Ave. Montreal, P.Q. H3A 1A1	514-842-1231	kidney heart lung heart-lung
	Maisonneuve-Rosemont 5415 boul. de L'Assomption Montreal, P.Q. H1T 2M4	514-252-3400	kidney
	Montreal General Hospital 1650 Cedar Ave. Montreal, P.Q. H3G 1A4	514-937-6011	kidney lung pancreas
	l'Hôpital Notre Dame 1560 rue Sherbrooke est Montreal, P.Q. H2L 4M1	514-876-6421	kidney liver pancreas heart
	l'Hôpital Ste-Justine 3175 chemin Ste-Catherine Montreal, P.Q. H3T 1C5	514-345-4931	kidney (pediatric) liver (pediatric) heart (pediatric)
	Montreal Cardiology Institute 5000 rue Belanger est Montreal, P.Q. H1T 1C8	514-376-3330	heart heart-lung
	Montreal Children's Hospital 2300 Tupper St. Montreal, P.Q. H3H 1P3	514-934-4400	heart (neonate) liver (pediatric)
	l'Hôpital St-Luc 1058 rue St-Denis Montreal, P.Q. H2X 3J4	514-281-2121	liver

	Centre Hospitalier-
	  Universitaire de
	  Sherbrooke
	375 Argyle St.
	Sherbrooke, P.Q.
	J1J 3H5
		819-563-5555	kidney

	Hôtel-Dieu de Québec 11 Côte du Palais Quebec City, P.Q. G1R 2J6	418-691-5151	kidney
Nova Scotia	Victoria General Hospital 1278 Tower Rd. Halifax, N.S. B3H 2Y9	902-428-2110	kidney liver heart
	Izaak Walton Killam Children's Hospital 5850 University Ave. Halifax, N.S. B3J 3G9	902-428-8111	kidney (pediatric)

U.S.
TRANSPLANT CENTERS

Children's Hospital of Alabama   205-939-9100
Division of Kidney Transplantation
1601 6th Ave. South
Birmingham, AL   35122

Baptist Medical Center — Princeton   205-783-3000
Division of Heart Transplantation
817 Princeton Ave. SW, #300
Birmingham, AL   35211

University of Alabama, Birmingham   205-934-4011
Division of Heart Transplantation
University Station
Birmingham, AL   35294

University of Arkansas Hospital   501-661-5000
Division of Kidney Transplantation
4301 W. Markham
Little Rock, AR   72201

Arkansas Children's Hospital   501-370-1100
Dept. of Nephrology
800 Marshall St.
Little Rock, AR   72202-3591

Good Samaritan Medical Center   602-239-2000
Division of Transplantation
1111 E. McDowell Rd., 925 Bldg.
Phoenix, AZ   85006

VA Hospitals   602-792-1450
Division of Kidney Transplantation
3601 S. 6th St.
Tucson, AZ   85723

Arizona Heart Institute   602-955-1000
Division of Heart Transplantation
P.O. Box 10,000
Phoenix, AZ   85064

University of Arizona   602-626-6000
Division of Heart Transplantation
Health Sciences Center, Room 4402
Tucson, AZ   85724

Children's Hospital of Los Angeles   213-660-2450
Division of Kidney Transplantation
4650 Sunset Blvd.
Los Angeles, CA   90027

San Bernadino County Medical Center   714-387-8111
Division of Kidney Transplantation
780 E. Gilbert St.
San Bernadino, CA   92404

Sharp Memorial Hospital   619-541-3400
Division of Heart Transplantation
7901 Frost St.
San Diego, CA   92123-2788

St. Joseph Hospital Hemodialysis Unit   714-633-9111
Division of Kidney Transplantation
1100 W. Stewart Dr.
Orange, CA   92668

St. Vincent Medical Center   213-484-5501
Division of Kidney Transplantation
2131 W. 3rd St.
Los Angeles, CA   90057

Sutter General Hospital   916-454-2222
Division of Transplantation
2820 L St.
Sacramento, CA   95816

University Hospital UCSD Medical Center   619-543-6222
Division of Kidney Transplantation
225 W. Dickenson St.
San Diego, CA   92103

University of California, San Francisco   415-476-1000
Division of Transplantation
UC Moffit, Room 884
San Francisco, CA   95817

University of California   714-634-6011
Irvine Medical Center
Division of Kidney Transplantation
101 City Drive South
Orange, CA   92668

Cedars Sinai Medical Center   213-855-5000
Division of Kidney Transplantation
8700 Beverly Blvd., Schuman Bldg., Room 635
Los Angeles, CA   90048

City of Hope National Medical Center   818-359-8111
Bone Marrow Transplant Program
1500 E. Duarte Rd.
Duarte, CA   91010

UCLA Hospital Center for Health Sciences   213-825-9111
Division of Transplantation
10833 LeConte Ave.
Los Angeles, CA   90024

University of California   916-453-2011
Davis Medical Center
Division of Transplantation
2315 Stockton Blvd.
Sacramento, CA   95817

Stanford University Medical Center   415-723-4000
Division of Heart Transplantation
Stanford, CA 94305

Los Angeles County USC Medical Center   213-226-2622
Division of Kidney Transplantation
1200 N. State St.
Los Angeles, CA   90033

Scripps Clinic and Research Foundation   619-455-9100
Weingart Center for Bone Marrow Transplantation
10666 N. Terry Pines Rd.
La Jolla, CA   92037

Santa Rosa Memorial Hospital   707-546-3210
Kidney Transplant Clinic
1154 Montgomery Dr., Suite 1
Santa Rosa, CA   95405

Pacific Medical Center — Presbyterian   415-563-4321
Division of Transplantation
P.O. Box 7999
San Francisco, CA   94120

Loma Linda University Medical Center   714-796-3741
Division of Transplantation
11234 Anderson St.
Loma Linda, CA   92354

Children's Hospital, San Diego   619-576-1700
Bone Marrow Transplant Program
8001 Frost St.
San Diego, CA   92123

Los Angeles County Harbor — UCLA Medical Center Division of Kidney Transplantation 1000 W. Carson St. Torrance, CA 90509	213-533-2345
Alta Bates Hospital Bone Marrow Transplant Program 3001 Colby St. Berkeley, CA 94705	415-540-0337
Samuel Merritt Hospital Division of Heart Transplantation 3300 Webster St., #304 Oakland, CA 94609	415-655-4000
Porter Memorial Hospital Dialysis Center Division of Kidney Transplantation 2525 S. Downing St. Denver, CO 80210	303-778-1955
St. Luke's Hospital Division of Transplantation 601 E. 19th Ave. Denver, CO 80203	303-839-1000
University of Colorado Health Sciences Center Division of Transplantation 4200 E. 9th Ave., Box C-310 Denver, CO 80262	303-399-1211
Hartford Hospital Division of Transplantation 80 Seymore St. Hartford, CT 06115	203-524-3011
Yale University School of Medicine Division of Heart Transplantation 333 Cedar St. New Haven, CT 06510	203-432-4771
Children's Hospital National Medical Center Division of Kidney Transplantation 111 Michigan Ave. NW Washington, DC 20010	202-745-5000
George Washington University Hospital Division of Kidney Transplantation 2150 Pennsylvania Ave. NW Washington, DC 20037	202-994-1000
Georgetown University Hospital Division of Kidney Transplantation 3800 Reservoir Rd. NW Washington, DC 20007	202-687-5055

Howard University Hospital
Division of Transplantation
2112 Georgia Ave. NW
Washington, DC   20060

202-865-6100

Washington Hospital Center
Division of Transplantation
110 Irving St. NW
Washington, DC   20010

202-877-7000

Vincent T. Lombardi Cancer Research Center
Bone Marrow Transplant Program
3800 Reservoir Rd. NW
Washington, DC   20007

202-687-2110

Florida Hospital
Division of Kidney Transplantation
601 E. Rollins Ave.
Orlando, FL   32803

407-896-6611

Jackson Memorial Hospital
Division of Kidney Transplantation
1611 NW 12th Ave.
Miami, FL   33136

305-325-7429

Shands Teaching Hospital and Clinics
Division of Transplantation
JHMHC Box J-223
Gainesville, FL   32610

904-395-0111

Tampa General Hospital
Division of Transplantation
Davis Island
Tampa, FL   33606

813-251-7443

Tallahassee Memorial Regional Center
Division of Heart Transplantation
1401 Centerville Rd., #803
Tallahassee, FL   32308

904-681-1155

Jackson Memorial Cardiac Transplant Center
Division of Heart Transplantation
School of Medicine, P.O. Box 01690
Miami, FL   33101

305-325-7429

All Children's Hospital
Bone Marrow Transplant Program
801 6th St. South
St. Petersburg, FL   33701

813-898-7451

University of Florida
Division of Transplantation
Box J-286, JHM Health Center
Gainesville, FL   32610

904-392-2623

Atlanta Regional Nephrology Center   404-589-4700
Division of Kidney Transplantation
80 Butler St. SE
Atlanta, GA   30303

Cardiothoracic Surgical Associates of Augusta   404-724-3568
Division of Heart Transplantation
820 S. Sebastian Way
Augusta, GA   30901-2690

Eugene Talmadge Memorial Hospital   404-721-0211
Medical College of Georgia
Division of Transplantation
1120 15th St.
Augusta, GA   30912

Henrietta Egleton Hospital for Children   404-325-6000
Division of Kidney Transplantation
1405 Clifton Rd. NE
Atlanta, GA   30322

Piedmont Hospital   404-350-2222
Division of Kidney Transplantation
105 Collier Rd.
Atlanta, GA   30309

St. Joseph's Hospital   404-851-7001
Division of Heart Transplantation
5665 Peach Tree Dunwoody Rd.
Atlanta, GA   30342

Emory Clinic   404-589-4307
Division of Transplantation
1364 Clifton Rd. NE
Atlanta, GA   30322

St. Francis Medical Office Bldg.   808-547-6011
Division of Heart Transplantation
2228 Liliha St., #208
Honolulu, HI   96817

Mercy Hospital Medical Center   515-247-3185
Division of Transplantation
6th St. & University Ave.
Des Moines, IA   50314

VA Hospital   319-338-0581
Division of Kidney Transplantation
Highway 6 W.
Iowa City, IA   52240

Mercy Hospital Medical Center   515-247-3185
Division of Heart Transplantation
6th St. & University Ave.
Des Moines, IA   50314

University of Iowa Hospitals and Clinics   319-356-1616
Division of Heart Transplantation
Iowa City, IA   52242

Children's Memorial Hospital   312-880-4000
Division of Kidney Transplantation
2300 Children's Plaza
Chicago, IL   60614

Memorial Medical Center   217-788-3000
Division of Kidney Transplantation
800 N. Rutledge St.
Springfield, IL   62781

St. Francis Medical Center   309-655-2000
Division of Kidney Transplantation
1124 N. Berkeley
Peoria, IL   61603

University of Illinois College of Medicine   312-996-3500
Division of Heart Transplantation
Box 6998
Chicago, IL   60680

Hines VA Hospital   312-343-7200
Division of Heart Transplantation
III-G
Hines, IL   60141

Loyola University Medical Center   312-531-3000
Division of Transplantation
2160 South First Ave.
Maywood, IL   60153

McGaw Medical Center   312-531-3000
Division of Heart Transplantation
2650 Ridge Ave.
Evanston, IL   60201

St. John's Hospital   217-544-6464
Bone Marrow Transplant Program
800 E. Carpenter St.
Springfield, IL   62769

Rush Presbyterian St. Luke's Medical Center   312-942-5492
Division of Transplantation
1753 W. Congress Pkwy, Room 1714 Jelke
Chicago, IL   60612

University of Chicago   312-702-1000
Division of Transplantation
5841 S. Maryland Ave.
Chicago, IL   60637

Downstate Heart Transplant Center   309-655-2000
Division of Heart Transplantation
530 NE Glen Oak Ave.
Peoria, IL   61637

Northwestern Memorial Hospital   312-908-2000
446 Wesley Pavilion
250 E. Superior
Chicago, IL   60611

Indiana University Hospitals   317-274-5000
Division of Transplantation
926 W. Michigan St., Room C-430
Indianapolis, IN   46223

St. Vincent Hospital and Health Care Center   317-871-2345
Division of Heart Transplantation
2001 W. 68th St., P.O. Box 40970
Indianapolis, IN   46240-0970

Lutheran Hospital of Ft. Wayne   219-458-2188
Division of Heart Transplantation
3024 Fairfield Ave.
Ft. Wayne, IN   46807

Methodist Hospital of Indiana   317-929-2000
Division of Heart Transplantation
1701 N. Senate Blvd.
Indianapolis, IN   46202

St. Francis Hospital   316-268-5000
Division of Transplantation
929 N. St. Francis Ave.
Wichita, KS   67214

University of Kansas Medical Center   913-588-5000
Division of Heart Transplantation
Kansas City, KS   66103

Kansas Heart Institute   913-233-1690
Division of Heart Transplantation
634 Mulvane St. #203
Topeka, KS   66606

Humana Heart Institute International   502-636-7135
Division of Heart Transplantation
One Audobon Plaza Drive
Louisville, KY   40217

Jewish Hospital   502-587-4011
Division of Transplantation
217 E. Chestnut St.
Louisville, KY   40202

University of Kentucky Medical Center   606-233-5000
Division of Transplantation
800 Rose St.
Lexington, KY   40536

Schumpert Medical Center   318-227-4500
Division of Kidney Transplantation
915 Margaret Place
Shreveport, LA   71120

Southern Baptist Hospital   504-899-9311
Division of Kidney Transplantation
2700 Napoleon Ave.
New Orleans, LA   70115

Tulane Medical Center   504-588-5263
Division of Transplantation
1430 Tulane Ave., Room 8700
New Orleans, LA   70113

Louisiana State University Medical Center   318-674-5000
Organ/Tissue Procurement
1501 Kingshighway
Shreveport, LA   71130

Oschner Clinic   504-838-4000
Division of Transplantation
1514 Jefferson Hwy
New Orleans, LA   70121

Hotel Dieu Hospital   504-588-3000
Division of Transplantation
2021 Perdido St.
New Orleans, LA   70112

Children's Hospital   617-735-6000
Division of Transplantation
300 Longwood Ave.
Boston, MA   02115

New England Deaconess Hospital   617-732-7000
Division of Transplantation
185 Pilgrim Rd.
Boston, MA   02215

University Hospital   617-638-8000
Division of Kidney Transplantation
75 E. Newton St.
Boston, MA   02118

Massachusetts General Hospital   617-726-2000
Division of Transplantation
Fruit St.
Boston, MA   02118

New England Medical Center Hospital   617-956-5000
Division of Transplantation
171 Harrison Ave.
Boston, MA   02111

Brigham and Women's Hospital   617-732-5500
Division of Transplantation
75 Francis St.
Boston, MA   02115

Dana Farber Cancer Institute   617-732-3000
Bone Marrow Transplant Program
44 Binney St.
Boston, MA   02115

New England Medical Center   617-956-5000
Division of Heart Transplantation
750 Washington St., Box 79
Boston, MA   02111

Beth Israel Hospital   617-735-2000
Renal Division
330 Brookline Ave.
Boston, MA   02215

Johns Hopkins Hospital   301-955-5000
Division of Transplantation
601 N. Broadway
Baltimore, MD   21205

University of Maryland Medical System   301-328-2121
Division of Transplantation
22 S. Greene St.
Baltimore, MD   21201

Francis Scott Key Medical Center   301-550-0100
4940 Eastern Ave.
Baltimore, MD   21224

Maine Medical Center   207-871-0111
Nephrology Department
22 Bramhall St.
Portland, ME   04102

Borgess Medical Center   616-383-7000
Division of Kidney Transplantation
1521 Gull Rd.
Kalamazoo, MI   49001

Hurley Medical Center   313-257-9000
Division of Kidney Transplantation
1 Hurley Plaza
Flint, MI   48502

Hutzel Hospital   313-745-7555
Division of Kidney Transplantation
4707 St-Antoine
Detroit, MI   48201

Mt. Carmel Mercy Hospital   313-927-7000
Division of Transplantation
6071 W. Outer Dr.
Detroit, MI   48235

St. Mary's Hospital   616-774-6090
Division of Kidney Transplantation
200 Jefferson St. SE
Grand Rapids, MI   49503

William Beaumont Hospital   313-288-7000
Division of Kidney Transplantation
3601 W. 13 Mile Rd.
Royal Oak, MI   48072

University of Michigan Medical School   313-936-4000
Bone Marrow Transplant Program
Mott Children's Hospital, F6515
Ann Arbor, MI   48109

Henry Ford Hospital   313-876-2600
Division of Heart Transplantation
2799 W. Grand Blvd.
Detroit, MI   48202

Children's Hospital of Michigan   313-745-5437
Division of Kidney Transplantation
3901 Beaubien St.
Detroit, MI   48201

University of Michigan Hospitals   313-936-4990
Division of Heart Transplantation
Taubman Health Care Center, 2110, Box 03
Ann Arbor, MI   48109

Regional Kidney Disease Program   612-347-5800
Division of Kidney Transplantation
825 S. 8th St.
Minneapolis, MN   55404

Rochester Methodist Hospital   507-286-7890
Division of Kidney Transplantation
201 W. Center St.
Rochester, MN   55901

Mayo Clinic   507-284-2511
Bone Marrow Transplant Program
Division of Hematology
Rochester, MN   55905

Abbott Northwestern Hospital
Division of Heart Transplantation
800 E. 28th St. at Chicago Ave.
Minneapolis, MN   55407

612-863-4000

Barnes Hospital
5300 Transplant Office
4949 Barnes Hospital Plaza
St. Louis, MO   63110

314-362-5000

Cardinal Glennon Memorial Hospital
Division of Kidney Transplantation
1465 S. Grand Blvd.
St. Louis, MO   63104

314-577-5600

Kansas City Dialysis and Transplant Center
Division of Kidney Transplantation
1734 E. 63rd St., #300
Kansas City, MO   64110

816-444-2098

Research Hospital and Medical Center
Division of Kidney Transplantation
2316 E. Meyer Bldg.
Kansas City, MO   64132

816-276-4000

St. Louis Children's Hospital
Division of Kidney Transplantation
500 S. Kingshighway Rd.
St. Louis, MO   63110

314-454-6000

St. Louis University Hospitals
Division of Transplantation
1325 S. Grand Blvd.
St. Louis, MO   63104

314-577-8000

St. Luke's Hospital
Division of Transplantation
P.O. Box 119000
Kansas City, MO   64111

816-932-2000

University of Missouri Hospital and Clinics
Division of Kidney Transplantation
One Hospital Dr.
Columbia, MO   65201

314-882-4141

VA Hospital
Division of Transplantation
915 North Grand St.
St. Louis, MO   63106

314-652-4100

Washington University School of Medicine
Division of Transplantation
4989 Barnes Hospital Plaza
St. Louis, MO   63110

314-362-5000

St. Luke's Hospital of Kansas City   816-932-2000
Division of Heart Transplantation
Wornall Rd. at 44th St.
Kansas City, MO   64111

University of Mississippi   601-984-1000
Mississippi Transplant Program
2500 N. State St.
Jackson, MS   39216

East Carolina School of Medicine   919-752-5480
Division of Heart Transplantation
Thoracic and Cardiovascular Surgery
Greenville, NC   27834

North Carolina Baptist Hospital   919-748-2011
Division of Kidney Transplantation
300 S. Hawthorn Rd.
Winston/Salem, NC   27103

North Carolina Memorial Hospital   919-966-4131
Division of Transplantation
Manning Drive, P.O. Box 501
Chapel Hill, NC   27514

Pitt County Memorial Hospital   919-551-4100
Division of Kidney Transplantation
Stantonsburg Rd., Box 6028
Greenville, NC   27834

Charlotte Memorial Hospital and
  Medical Center   704-338-2000
Division of Heart Transplantation
P.O. Box 32861
Charlotte, NC   28232

Duke Medical Center   919-752-5480
Division of Heart Transplantation
Box 3235
Durham, NC   27710

St. Joseph's Hospital   402-449-4000
Division of Kidney Transplantation
601 N. 30th St.
Omaha, NE   68131

University of Nebraska Medical Center   402-559-4000
Bone Marrow Transplant Unit
42nd St. & Dewey Ave.
Omaha, NE   68105

Bishop Clarkson Memorial Hospital   402-559-2000
Division of Transplantation
Dewey Ave. at 44th St.
Omaha, NE   68105

Bryan Memorial Hospital   402-489-0200
Division of Heart Transplantation
1600 S. 48th St.
Lincoln, NE   68506-1299

Our Lady of Lourdes Medical Center   609-757-3500
Division of Kidney Transplantation
1600 Haddon Ave.
Camden, NJ   08103

St. Barnabus Medical Center   201-533-5000
Division of Transplantation
Old Short Hills Rd.
Livingston, NJ   07039

Dialysis Clinic Inc.   505-243-1906
Division of Kidney Transplantation
1511 Central Ave. NE
Albuquerque, NM   87106

Presbyterian Transplant Center   505-841-1234
Division of Transplantation
1100 Central Ave. SE
Albuquerque, NM   87102

University of New Mexico Hospital   505-843-2111
Division of Kidney Transplantation
2211 Lomas Blvd. NE
Albuquerque, NM   87106

Albany Medical Center Hospital   518-445-3125
Division of Kidney Transplantation
New Scotland Ave.
Albany, NY   12208

Children's Hospital   716-878-7000
Division of Kidney Transplantation
219 Bryant St.
Buffalo, NY   14222

Downstate Medical Center   718-270-1000
Division of Kidney Transplantation
445 Lenox Rd., Box 23
Brooklyn, NY   11203

Erie County Medical Center   716-898-3000
Division of Kidney Transplantation
462 Grider St.
Buffalo, NY   14215

Montefiore Hospital   212-920-4321
Division of Transplantation
111 E. 210th St.
Bronx, NY   10467

New York Hospital   212-746-5454
Division of Kidney Transplantation
525 E. 68th St.
New York, NY   10021

Presbyterian Hospital   212-305-2500
Division of Transplantation
622 W. 168th St.
New York, NY   10032

Roswell Park Memorial Institute   716-845-2300
Bone Marrow Transplant Program
666 Elm St.
Buffalo, NY   14263

St. Luke's Hospital Center   212-523-4000
Division of Kidney Transplantation
Amsterdam Ave. & 114th St.
New York, NY   10025

State University Hospital Upstate
   Medical Center   315-473-5540
Division of Kidney Transplantation
750 E. Adams St.
Syracuse, NY   13210

Strong Memorial Hospital — ESRD   716-275-2121
Division of Kidney Transplantation
601 Elmwood Ave.
Rochester, NY   14642

University Hospital Health Science Center   516-689-6000
Division of Kidney Transplantation
State University of New York
Stoney Brook, NY   11794

New York Medical College   914-993-4000
Bone Marrow Transplant Program
Division of Oncology
Valhalla, NY   10595

Buffalo General Hospital   716-845-5600
Division of Transplantation
100 High St.
Buffalo, NY   14203

Mt. Sinai Medical Center   212-241-6500
Division of Transplantation
One Gustave L. Levy Plaza
New York, NY   10029

Columbia Presbyterian Medical Center   212-305-2500
Division of Heart Transplantation
622 W. 168th St.
New York, NY   10032

Memorial Sloane Kettering   212-794-7722
Bone Marrow Transplant Program
1275 York Ave.
New York, NY   11021

Case Western Reserve, University Hospital   216-844-1000
Bone Marrow Transplant Program
University Circle
Cleveland, OH   44106

Children's Hospital — ESRD   614-461-2000
Division of Kidney Transplantation
700 Children's Dr.
Columbus, OH   43205

Children's Hospital Medical Center   216-379-8200
Division of Kidney Transplantation
281 Locust St.
Akron, OH   44308

Christ Hospital   513-369-2000
Division of Kidney Transplantation
2139 Auburn St.
Cincinnati, OH   45219

Medical College of Ohio at Toledo   419-381-4172
Division of Kidney Transplantation
3000 Arlington Ave., CS 10008
Toledo, OH   43699

Miami Valley Hospital   513-223-6192
Division of Kidney Transplantation
One Wyoming St.
Dayton, OH   45409

Ohio State University Hospitals   614-293-8000
Division of Transplantation
410 W. 10th Ave.
Columbus, OH   43210

University Hospital   513-558-1000
Division of Transplantation
234 Goodman St.
Cincinnati, OH   45267

Cleveland Clinic Foundation, A-72   216-444-2200
Dept. of Allergy and Immunology
9500 Euclid Ave.
Cleveland, OH   44106

University Hospital of Cleveland   216-844-1000
Division of Kidney Transplantation
2074 Abington Rd.
Cleveland, OH   44106

University of Cincinnati   513-558-5111
Division of Transplantation
231 Bethesda Ave. (ML558)
Cincinnati, OH   45267-0558

University of Cincinnati Medical Center   513-558-1000
231 Bethesda Ave.
Cincinnati, OH   45267-0585

Medical College of Ohio   419-381-4172
C.S. 10008
Toledo, OH   43699

Cleveland Clinic Foundation   216-444-2200
Division of Transplantation
9500 Euclid Ave.
Cleveland, OH   44106

Akron City Hospital   216-375-3000
Division of Kidney Transplantation
525 E. Market St.
Akron, OH   44309

Baptist Medical Center of Oklahoma   405-949-3011
Division of Transplantation
3300 NW Expressway
Oklahoma City, OK   73112

Hillcrest Medical Center   918-584-1351
Division of Kidney Transplantation
1145 S. Utica Ave., Ste. 607
Tulsa, OK   74104

Oklahoma Children's Memorial Hospital   405-271-4371
Division of Kidney Transplantation
P.O. Box 26901
Oklahoma City, OK   73190

Oklahoma Memorial Hospital   405-271-4700
Division of Kidney Transplantation
P.O. Box 26307
Oklahoma City, OK   73126

University of Oklahoma   405-271-2339
Bone Marrow Transplant Program
Dept. of Medicine, Section of Oncology
Oklahoma City, OK   73190

St. Anthony Hospital   405-272-7000
Division of Heart Transplantation
1000 North Lee St.
Oklahoma City, OK   73101

Oregon Health Sciences University   503-279-8311
Division of Transplantation
3181 SW Sam Jackson Park Rd.
Portland, OR   97201

Albert Einstein Medical Center   215-456-7890
Division of Kidney Transplantation
York & Tabor Rds
Philadelphia, PA   19141

Geisinger Medical Center   717-271-6211
Division of Kidney Transplantation
N. Academy Ave.
Danville, PA   17822

Hahnemann University Hospital   215-448-7000
Division of Transplantation
230 N. Broad St.
Philadelphia, PA   19102

Presbyterian University Hospital   412-647-2345
Division of Transplantation
Desoto at O'Hara Sts
Pittsburgh, PA   15213

Thomas Jefferson University Hospital   215-928-6000
Division of Transplantation
11 Walnut St.
Philadelphia, PA   19107

University of Pennsylvania Hospital   215-662-4000
Division of Transplantation
34th & Spruce Sts
Philadelphia, PA   19104

Children's Hospital of Philadelphia   215-596-9100
Bone Marrow Transplant Program
34th & Civic Center Blvd.
Philadelphia, PA   19104

Milton Hershey Medical Center   215-531-8521
Division of Heart Transplantation
Dept. of Surgery, P.O. Box 850
Hershey, PA   17033

Temple University Hospital   215-221-2000
Division of Heart Transplantation
3401 North Broad St.
Philadelphia, PA   19140

Children's Hospital of Pittsburgh   412-647-5325
One Children's Place
705 Fifth Ave. at DeSoto St.
Pittsburgh, PA   15213

University of Pittsburgh   412-647-2345
Division of Heart Transplantation
1088 Sciafe Hall
Pittsburgh, PA   15261

Allegheny General Hospital   412-359-3131
320 East North Ave.
Pittsburgh, PA   15261

Montefiore Hospital   412-648-6000
Bone Marrow Transplant Program
3459 5th Ave.
Pittsburgh, PA   15213

St. Christopher's Hospital for Children   215-427-5000
Pediatric Heart Institute
5th & Lehigh Ave.
Philadelphia, PA   19133

Auxilio Mutuo Hospital   809-764-1488
Division of Kidney Transplantation
Ponce De Leon Ave.
Hato Pey, PR   00919

MUSC Hemo and Transplant Program   803-792-2300
Division of Transplantation
171 Ashley Ave.
Charleston, SC   29425-2279

Le Bonheur Children's Hospital   901-522-3000
Division of Transplantation
848 Adams Ave.
Memphis, TN   38103

University of Tennessee   615-974-1000
Division of Kidney Transplantation
1924 Alcoa Hwy
Knoxville, TN   37920

University of Tennessee Medical Center   901-577-4000
Division of Transplantation
956 Court
Memphis, TN   38163

St. Thomas Hospital   615-386-2111
Division of Heart Transplantation
4220 Harding Rd., P.O. Box 380
Nashville, TN   37202

Vanderbilt University   615-322-7311
Division of Transplantation
1211 21st Ave. S., #338
Nashville, TN   37212

Brackenridge Hospital   512-459-1111
Division of Kidney Transplantation
15th St. & East Ave.
Austin, TX   78701

Children's Medical Center — ESRD   214-920-2000
Division of Transplantation
1935 Motor St.
Dallas, TX   75235

Hermann Hospital   713-797-4011
Division of Transplantation
1203 Ross Sterling Ave.
Houston, TX   77025

Humana Hospital   512-692-8110
Division of Kidney Transplantation
8026 Floyd Curl Dr.
San Antonio, TX   78229

Lubbock General Hospital Organ   806-743-3111
    Procurement Agency
602 Indiana Ave., Box 5980
Lubbock, TX   79417

Medical Center Hospital   512-694-3030
Division of Kidney Transplantation
4502 Medical Dr.
San Antonio, TX   78284

Methodist Hospital   713-790-3311
Division of Transplantation
6516 Bertner Blvd.
Houston, TX   77025

Methodist Medical Center   214-944-8181
Division of Transplantation
301 W. Colorado Blvd.
Dallas, TX   75208

Parkland Memorial Hospital   214-590-8000
Division of Kidney Transplantation
5201 Harry Hines Blvd.
Dallas, TX   75235

St. Luke's Episcopal Hospital   713-791-2011
Division of Transplantation
6720 Bertner St.
Houston, TX   77030

Texas Heart Institute   409-791-4011
Division of Heart Transplantation
P.O. Box 20269
Houston, TX   77225

University of Texas Medical Branch   409-761-1011
Division of Transplantation
Old John Sealy Hospital
Galveston, TX   77550

Anderson Hospital and Tumer Institute   713-792-2121
1515 Holcombe Blvd.
Houston, TX   77030

Baylor College of Medicine   713-798-4951
Bone Marrow Transplant Program
6565 Fannin St., MS 902
Houston, TX   77030

Baylor University Medical Center   214-820–0111
Division of Transplantation
3500 Gaston Ave.
Dallas, TX   75246

St. Paul Medical Center   214-879-1000
Division of Heart Transplantation
Dallas, TX   75235

University of Texas Health Science Center   512-567-7000
Bone Marrow Transplant Program
7703 Floyd Curl St.
San Antonio, TX   78284

Children's Medical Center   817-885-4000
Transplant Services
1212 W. Lancaster Ave.
Fort Worth, TX   76102

Seton Medical Center   512-459-2121
Division of Heart Transplantation
1201 W. 38th St.
Austin, TX   78705-1056

Harris Hospital — Methodist   817-882-2000
Division of Kidney Transplantation
1300 W. Cannon
Fort Worth, TX   76104

Methodist Hospital   713-790-3311
Division of Heart Transplantation
6535 Fannin, MS F-1001
Houston, TX   77030

Latter Day Saints Hospital   801-321-1100
Division of Transplantation
325 8th Ave.
Salt Lake City, UT   84143

VA Hospital   801-582-1565
Division of Transplantation
500 Foothill Dr.
Salt Lake City, UT   84148

University of Utah Medical Center   801-581-2121
Division of Transplantation
50 N. Medical Dr.
Salt Lake City, UT   84132

Norfolk General Hospital — ESRD   804-628-3000
Division of Kidney Transplantation
600 Gresham Dr.
Norfolk, VA   23507

University of Virginia Hospital   804-924-5161
Division of Kidney Transplantation
University Station, Box 133
Charlottesville, VA   22908

Virginia Cardiovascular Surgery Associates, PC   703-280-5858
Division of Heart Transplantation
3301 Woodburn Rd., #301
Fairfax, VA   22003

McGuire VA Medical Center   804-230-0001
Division of Transplantation
1200 Broad Rock Blvd.
Richmond, VA   23249

Medical College of Virginia   804-786-9000
Box 499 MCV Station
Richmond, VA   23298-0499

Medical Center Hospital of Vermont   802-656-2345
Division of Kidney Transplantation
Colchester Ave.
Burlington, VT   05401

Children's Orthopaedic Hospital   206-526-2000
Division of Kidney Transplantation
4800 Sand Point Way NE
Seattle, WA   98105

Sacred Heart Medical Center   509-455-3131
Division of Transplantation and
   Organ Procurement
W. 101 8th Ave.
Spokane, WA   99220

Swedish Hospital Medical Center   206-386-6000
Division of Kidney Transplantation
747 Summit Ave.
Seattle, WA   98104

University Hospital   206-548-3300
Division of Transplantation
1959 E. Pacific St., RF-25
Seattle, WA   98195

Virginia Mason Hospital   206-624-1144
Division of Kidney Transplantation
925 Senaca St.
Seattle, WA   98101

University of Washington   206-543-2100
Division of Heart Transplantation
Dept. of Surgery, RF-25
Seattle, WA   98195

VA Medical Center   206-762-1010
Bone Marrow Transplant Program
1660 S. Columbian Way
Seattle, WA   90108

Fred Hutchinson Cancer Research Center   206-467-5000
Bone Marrow Transplant Program
1124 Columbia St.
Seattle, WA   98104

Froedtert Memorial Lutheran Hospital   414-259-3000
Division of Transplantation
9200 W. Wisconsin Ave.
Milwaukee, WI   53226

University of Wisconsin Hospital and Clinics   608-263-6400
Division of Transplantation
600 Highland Ave.
Madison, WI   53792

Marshfield Clinic   715-387-5511
Bone Marrow Transplant Program
1000 N. Oak Ave.
Marshfield, WI   54449

University of Wisconsin   608-263-6400
Bone Marrow Transplant Program
1300 University Ave.
Madison, WI   53706

Medical College of Wisconsin   414-257-8296
Division of Heart Transplantation
Milwaukee County Medical Complex
Milwaukee, WI   53201

Midwest Heart Surgery Ltd.   414-647-1120
Division of Heart Transplantation
2901 W. Kinnickinnic River Pkwy
Milwaukee, WI   53215

HUMAN TISSUE GIFT ACT, 1986 ONTARIO MINISTRY OF THE SOLICITOR GENERAL

Author's note: All provinces and territories have some organ donation legislation similar to the following Ontario Act. In Quebec, organ donation legislation falls under the Civil Code. Manitoba is the only province to have legislated "required consideration." Physicians are required to consider patients who have died as potential donors. If a potential donor is identified, a staff member is to request permission from next of kin.

1. In this Act,

> (a) "consent" means a consent given under this Act;
> (b) "physician" means a person licensed under Part III of the *Health Disciplines Act*;
> (c) "tissue" includes an organ, but does not include any skin, bone, blood, blood constituent or other tissue that is replaceable by natural processes of repair;
> (d) "transplant" as a noun means the removal of tissue from a human body, whether living or dead, and its implantation in a living human body, and in its other forms it has corresponding meanings;
> (e) "writing" for the purposes of Part II includes a will and any other testamentary instrument whether or not probate has been applied for or granted and whether or not the will or other testamentary instrument is valid.   R.S.O. 1980, c. 210, s. 1.

PART I: *INTER-VIVOS* GIFTS FOR TRANSPLANTS

2. A transplant from one living human body to another living human body may be done in accordance with this Act, but not otherwise. R.S.O. 1980, c. 210, s. 2.

3. — (1) Any person who has attained the age of sixteen years, is mentally competent to consent, and is able to make a free and informed decision may in a writing signed by him consent to the removal forthwith from his body of the tissue specified in the consent and its implantation in the body of another living person. R.S.O. 1980, c. 210, s. 3 (1); 1986, c. 64, s. 19 (1).

(2) Notwithstanding subsection (1), a consent given there-under by a person who had not attained the age of sixteen years, was not mentally competent to consent, or was not able to make a free and informed decision is valid for the purposes of this Act if the person who acted upon it had no reason to believe that the person who gave it had not attained the age of sixteen years, was not mentally competent to consent, and was not able to make a free and informed decision, as the case may be. R.S.O. 1980, c. 210, s. 3 (2); 1986, c. 64, s. 19 (2).

(3) A consent given under this section is full authority for any physician,

    (a) to make any examination necessary to assure medical acceptability of the tissue specified therein; and

    (b) to remove forthwith such tissue from the body of the person who gave the consent.

(4) If for any reason the tissue specified in the consent is not removed in the circumstances to which the consent relates, the consent is void. R.S.O. 1980, c. 210, s. 3 (3, 4).

PART II   *POST MORTEM* GIFTS FOR TRANSPLANTS AND OTHER USES

4. — (1) Any person who has attained the age of sixteen years may consent,

    (a) in a writing signed by him at any time; or

    (b) orally in the presence of at least two witnesses during his last illness,

that his body or the part or parts thereof specified in the consent be used after his death for therapeutic purposes, medical education or scientific research. R.S.O. 1980, c. 210, s. 4 (1); 1986, c. 64, s. 19 (3).

(2) Notwithstanding subsection (1), a consent given by a person who had not attained the age of sixteen years is valid for the purposes of this Act if the person who acted upon it had no reason to believe that the person who gave it had not attained the age of sixteen years. R.S.O. 1980, c. 210, s. 4 (2); 1986, c. 64, s. 19 (4).

(3)   Upon the death of a person who has given a consent under this section, the consent is binding and is full authority for the use of the body or the removal and use of the specified part or parts for the purpose specified, except that no person shall act upon a consent given under this section if he has reason to believe that it was subsequently withdrawn.   R.S.O. 1980, c. 210, s. 4 (3).

5. — (1)   In this section, "spouse" means a person of the opposite sex,

    (a)   to whom the person is married; or

    (b)   with whom the person is living or, immediately before the person's death, was living in a conjugal relationship outside marriage, if the two persons,

        (i)   have cohabited for at least one year,

        (ii)   are together the parents of a child, or

        (iii)   have together entered into a cohabitation agreement under section 53 of the *Family Law Act, 1986.*

(1a)   Where a person who has not given or cannot give a consent under section 4 dies, or in the opinion of a physician is incapable of giving a consent by reason of injury or disease and the person's death is imminent,

    (a)   the person's spouse; or

    (b)   if none or if the spouse is not readily available, any one of the person's children; or

    (c)   if none or if none is readily available, either one of the person's parents; or

    (d)   if none or if neither is readily available, any one of the person's brothers or sisters; or

    (e)   if none or if none is readily available, any other of the person's next of kin; or

    (f)   if none or if none is readily available, the person lawfully in possession of the body other than, where the person died in hospital, the administrative head of the hospital,

may consent,

    (g)   in a writing signed by the spouse, relative or other person; or

    (h)   orally by the spouse, relative or other person in the presence of at least two witnesses; or

    (i)   by the telegraphic, recorded telephonic, or other recorded message of the spouse, relative or other person,

to the body or the part or parts thereof specified in the consent being used after death for therapeutic purposes, medical education or scientific research. 1986, c. 64, s. 19 (5).

(2)   No person shall give a consent under this section if he has reason to

believe that the person who died or whose death is imminent would have objected thereto.

(3) Upon the death of a person in respect of whom a consent was given under this section the consent is binding and is, subject to section 6, full authority for the use of the body or for the removal and use of the specified part or parts for the purpose specified except that no person shall act on a consent given under this section if he has actual knowledge of an objection thereto by the person in respect of whom the consent was given or by a person of the same or closer relationship to the person in respect of whom the consent was given than the person who gave the consent.

(4) In subsection (1), "person lawfully in possession of the body" does not include,

    (a)   the Chief Coroner or a coroner in possession of the body for the purposes of the *Coroners Act;*

    (b)   the Public Trustee in possession of the body for the purpose of its burial under the *Crown Administration of Estates Act;*

    (c)   an embalmer or funeral director in possession of the body for the purpose of its burial, cremation or other disposition; or

    (d)   the superintendent of a crematorium in possession of the body for the purpose of its cremation. R.S.O. 1980, c. 210, s. 5 (2-4).

6. Where, in the opinion of a physician, the death of a person is imminent by reason of injury or disease and the physician has reason to believe that section 10 of the *Coroners Act* may apply when death does occur and a consent under this Part has been obtained for a *post mortem* transplant of tissue from the body, a coroner having jurisdiction, notwithstanding that death has not yet occurred, may give such directions as he thinks proper respecting the removal of such tissue after the death of the person, and every such direction has the same force and effect as if it had been made after death under section 11 of the *Coroners Act.* R.S.O. 1980, c. 210, s. 6.

7. — (1) For the purposes of a *post mortem* transplant, the fact of death shall be determined by at least two physicians in accordance with accepted medical practice.

(2) No physician who has had any association with the proposed recipient that might influence his judgment shall take any part in the determination of the fact of death of the donor.

(3) No physician who took any part in the determination of the fact of death of the donor shall participate in any way in the transplant procedures.

(4) Nothing in this section in any way affects a physician in the removal of eyes for cornea transplants. R.S.O. 1980, c. 210, s. 7.

8. Where a gift under this Part cannot for any reason be used for any of the purposes specified in the consent, the subject-matter of the gift and the body to which it belongs shall be dealt with and disposed of as if no consent had been given. R.S.O. 1980, c. 210, s. 8.

PART III   GENERAL

9. No action or other proceeding for damages lies against any person for any act done in good faith and without negligence in the exercise or intended exercise of any authority conferred by this Act.   R.S.O. 1980, c. 210, s. 9.

10. No person shall buy, sell or otherwise deal in, directly or indirectly, for a valuable consideration, any tissue for a transplant, or any body or part or parts thereof other than blood or a blood constituent, for therapeutic purposes, medical education or scientific research, and any such dealing is invalid as being contrary to public policy.   R.S.O. 1980, c. 210, s. 10.

11. — (1)   Except where legally required, no person shall disclose or give to any other person any information or document whereby the identity of any person,

    (a)   who has given or refused to give a consent;

    (b)   with respect to whom a consent has been given; or

    (c)   into whose body tissue has been, is being or may be transplanted,

may become known publicly.

(2)   Where the information or document disclosed or given pertains only to the person who disclosed or gave the information or document, subsection (1) does not apply.   R.S.O. 1980, c. 210, s. 11.

12. Every person who knowingly contravenes any provision of this Act is guilty of an offence and on conviction is liable to a fine of not more than $1,000 or to imprisonment for a term of not more than six months, or to both. R.S.O. 1980, c. 210, s. 12.

13. Except as provided in section 6, nothing in this Act affects the operation of the *Coroners Act*.   R.S.O. 1980, c. 210, s. 13.

UNIFORM ANATOMICAL GIFT ACT (United States, 1987)

SECTION 1. DEFINITIONS.

As used in this [Act]:

(1) *"Anatomical gift"* means a donation of all or part of a human body to take effect upon or after death.

(2) *"Decedent"* means a deceased individual and includes a stillborn infant or fetus.

(3) *"Document of gift"* means a card, a statement attached to or imprinted on a motor vehicle operator's or chauffeur's license, a will, or other writing used to make an anatomical gift.

(4) *"Donor"* means an individual who makes an anatomical gift of all or part of the individual's body.

(5) *"Enucleator"* means an individual who is [licensed] [certified] by the [State Board of Medical Examiners] to remove or process eyes or parts of eyes.

(6) *"Hospital"* means a facility licensed, accredited, or approved as a hospital under the law of any state or a facility operated as a hospital by the United States government, a state, or a subdivision of a state.

(7) *"Part"* means an organ, tissue, eye, bone, artery, blood, fluid, or other portion of a human body.

(8) *"Person"* means an individual, corporation, business trust, estate, trust, partnership, joint venture, association, government, governmental subdivision or agency, or any other legal or commercial entity.

(9) *"Physician"* or *"surgeon"* means an individual licensed or otherwise authorized to practice medicine and surgery or osteopathy and surgery under the laws of any state.

(10) *"Procurement organization"* means a person licensed, accredited, or approved under the laws of any state for procurement, distribution, or storage of human bodies or parts.

(11)   "*State*" means a state, territory, or possession of the United States, the District of Columbia, or the Commonwealth of Puerto Rico.

(12)   "*Technician*" means an individual who is [licensed] [certified] by the [State Board of Medical Examiners] to remove or process a part.

SECTION 2.   MAKING, AMENDING, REVOKING, AND REFUSING TO MAKE ANATOMICAL GIFTS BY INDIVIDUAL.

(a)   An individual who is at least [18] years of age may (i) make an anatomical gift for any of the purposes stated in Section 6(a), (ii) limit an anatomical gift to one or more of those purposes, or (iii) refuse to make an anatomical gift.

(b)   An anatomical gift may be made only by a document of gift signed by the donor. If the donor cannot sign, the document of gift must be signed by another individual and by two witnesses, all of whom have signed at the direction and in the presence of the donor and of each other, and state that it has been so signed.

(c)   If a document of gift is attached to or imprinted on a donor's motor vehicle operator's or chauffeur's license, the document of gift must comply with subsection (b). Revocation, suspension, expiration, or cancellation of the license does not invalidate the anatomical gift.

(d)   A document of gift may designate a particular physician or surgeon to carry out the appropriate procedures. In the absence of a designation or if the designee is not available, the donee or other person authorized to accept the anatomical gift may employ or authorize any physician, surgeon, technician, or enucleator to carry out the appropriate procedures.

(e)   An anatomical gift by will takes effect upon death of the testator, whether or not the will is probated. If, after death, the will is declared invalid for testamentary purposes, the validity of the anatomical gift is unaffected.

(f)   A donor may amend or revoke an anatomical gift, not made by will, only by:

(1)   a signed statement;
(2)   an oral statement made in the presence of two individuals;
(3)   any form of communication during a terminal illness or injury addressed to a physician or surgeon; or
(4)   the delivery of a signed statement to a specified donee to whom a document of gift had been delivered.

(g)   The donor of an anatomical gift made by will may amend or revoke the gift in the manner provided for amendment or revocation of wills, or as provided in subsection (f).

(h)   An anatomical gift that is not revoked by the donor before death is irrevocable and does not require the consent or concurrence of any person after the donor's death.

(i) An individual may refuse to make an anatomical gift of the individual's body or part by (i) a writing signed in the same manner as a document of gift, (ii) a statement attached to or imprinted on a donor's motor vehicle operator's or chauffeur's license, or (iii) any other writing used to identify the individual as refusing to make an anatomical gift. During a terminal illness or injury, the refusal may be an oral statement or other form of communication.

(j) In the absence of contrary indications by the donor, an anatomical gift of a part is neither a refusal to give other parts nor a limitation on an anatomical gift under Section 3 or on a removal or release of other parts under Section 4.

(k) In the absence of contrary indications by the donor, a revocation or amendment of an anatomical gift is not a refusal to make another anatomical gift. If the donor intends a revocation to be a refusal to make an anatomical gift, the donor shall make the refusal pursuant to subsection (i).

SECTION 3. MAKING, REVOKING, AND OBJECTING TO ANATOMICAL GIFTS, BY OTHERS.

(a) Any member of the following classes of persons, in the order of priority listed, may make an anatomical gift of all or a part of the decedent's body for an authorized purpose, unless the decedent, at the time of death, has made an unrevoked refusal to make that anatomical gift:

(1) the spouse of the decedent;
(2) an adult son or daughter of the decedent;
(3) either parent of the decedent;
(4) an adult brother or sister of the decedent;
(5) a grandparent of the decedent; and
(6) a guardian of the person of the decedent at the time of death.

(b) An anatomical gift may not be made by a person listed in subsection (a) if:

(1) a person in a prior class is available at the time of death to make an anatomical gift;
(2) the person proposing to make an anatomical gift knows of a refusal or contrary indications by the decedent; or
(3) the person proposing to make an anatomical gift knows of an objection to making an anatomical gift by a member of the person's class or a prior class.

(c) An anatomical gift by a person authorized under subsection (a) must be made by (i) a document of gift signed by the person or (ii) the person's telegraphic, recorded telephonic, or other recorded message, or other form of communication from the person that is contemporaneously reduced to writing and signed by the recipient.

(d)   An anatomical gift by a person authorized under subsection (a) may be revoked by any member of the same or a prior class if, before procedures have begun for the removal of a part from the body of the decedent, the physician, surgeon, technician, or enucleator removing the part knows of the revocation.

(e)   A failure to make an anatomical gift under subsection (a) is not an objection to the making of an anatomical gift.

SECTION 4. AUTHORIZATION BY [CORONER] [MEDICAL EXAMINER] OR [LOCAL PUBLIC HEALTH OFFICIAL].

(a)   The [coroner] [medical examiner] may release and permit the removal of a part from a body within that official's custody, for transplantation or therapy, if:

> (1)   the official has received a request for the part from a hospital, physician, surgeon, or procurement organization;
>
> (2)   the official has made a reasonable effort, taking into account the useful life of the part, to locate and examine the decedent's medical records and inform persons listed in Section 3(a) of their option to make, or object to making, an anatomical gift;
>
> (3)   the official does not know of a refusal or contrary indication by the decedent or objection by a person having priority to act as listed in Section 3(a);
>
> (4)   the removal will be by a physician, surgeon, or technician; but in the case of eyes, by one of them or by an enucleator;
>
> (5)   the removal will not interfere with any autopsy or investigation;
>
> (6)   the removal will be in accordance with accepted medical standards; and
>
> (7)   cosmetic restoration will be done, if appropriate.

(b)   If the body is not within the custody of the [coroner] [medical examiner], the [local public health officer] may release and permit the removal of any part from a body in the [local public health officer's] custody for transplantation or therapy if the requirements of subsection (a) are met.

(c)   An official releasing and permitting the removal of a part shall maintain a permanent record of the name of the decedent, the person making the request, the date and purpose of the request, the part requested, and the person to whom it was released.

SECTION 5. ROUTINE INQUIRY AND REQUIRED REQUEST; SEARCH AND NOTIFICATION.

(a)   On or before admission to a hospital, or as soon as possible thereafter, a person designated by the hospital shall ask each patient who is at least [18] years of age: "Are you an organ or tissue donor?" If the answer is affirmative the person shall request a copy of the document of gift. If the answer is negative or there is no answer and the attending physician consents, the person designated shall discuss with the patient the option to make or refuse to make an anatomical gift. The answer to the question, an available copy of any document of gift or refusal to make an anatomical gift, and any other relevant information, must be placed in the patient's medical record.

(b) If, at or near the time of death of a patient, there is no medical record that the patient has made or refused to make an anatomical gift, the hospital [administrator] or a representative designated by the [administrator] shall discuss the option to make or refuse to make an anatomical gift and request the making of an anatomical gift pursuant to Section 3(a). The request must be made with reasonable discretion and sensitivity to the circumstances of the family. A request is not required if the gift is not suitable, based upon accepted medical standards, for a purpose specified in Section 6. An entry must be made in the medical record of the patient, stating the name and affiliation of the individual making the request, and of the name, response, and relationship to the patient of the person to whom the request was made. The [Commissioner of Health] shall [establish guidelines] [adopt regulations] to implement this subsection.

(c) The following persons shall make a reasonable search for a document of gift or other information identifying the bearer as a donor or as an individual who has refused to make an anatomical gift:

(1) a law enforcement officer, fireman, paramedic, or other emergency rescuer finding an individual who the searcher believes is dead or near death; and

(2) a hospital, upon the admission of an individual at or near the time of death, if there is not immediately available any other source of that information.

(d) If a document of gift or evidence of refusal to make an anatomical gift is located by the search required by subsection (c)(1), and the individual or body to whom it relates is taken to a hospital, the hospital must be notified of the contents and the document or other evidence must be sent to the hospital.

(e) If, at or near the time of death of a patient, a hospital knows that an anatomical gift has been made pursuant to Section 3(a) or a release and removal of a part has been permitted pursuant to Section 4, or that a patient or an individual identified as in transit to the hospital is a donor, the hospital shall notify the donee if one is named and known to the hospital; if not, it shall notify an appropriate procurement organization. The hospital shall cooperate in the implementation of the anatomical gift or release and removal of a part.

(f) A person who fails to discharge the duties imposed by this section is not subject to criminal or civil liability but is subject to appropriate administrative sanctions.

SECTION 6. PERSONS WHO MAY BECOME DONEES; PURPOSES FOR WHICH ANATOMICAL GIFTS MAY BE MADE.

(a)   The following persons may become donees of anatomical gifts for the purposes stated:

(1)   a hospital, physician, surgeon, or procurement organization, for transplantation, therapy, medical or dental education, research, or advancement of medical or dental science;

(2)   an accredited medical or dental school, college, or university for education, research, advancement of medical or dental science; or

(3)   a designated individual for transplantation or therapy needed by that individual.

(b)   An anatomical gift may be made to a designated donee or without designating a donee. If a donee is not designated or if the donee is not available or rejects the anatomical gift, the anatomical gift may be accepted by any hospital.

(c)   If the donee knows of the decedent's refusal or contrary indications to make an anatomical gift or that an anatomical gift by a member of a class having priority to act is opposed by a member of the same class or a prior class under Section 3(a), the donee may not accept the anatomical gift.

SECTION 7. DELIVERY OF DOCUMENT OF GIFT.

(a)   Delivery of a document of gift during the donor's lifetime is not required for the validity of an anatomical gift.

(b)   If an anatomical gift is made to a designated donee, the document of gift, or a copy, may be delivered to the donee to expedite the appropriate procedures after death. The document of gift, or a copy, may be deposited in any hospital, procurement organization, or registry office that accepts it for safekeeping or for facilitation of procedures after death. On request of an interested person, upon or after the donor's death, the person in possession shall allow the interested person to examine or copy the document of gift.

SECTION 8. RIGHTS AND DUTIES AT DEATH.

(a)   Rights of a donee created by an anatomical gift are superior to rights of others except with respect to autopsies under Section 11(b). A donee may accept or reject an anatomical gift. If a donee accepts an anatomical gift of an entire body, the donee, subject to the terms of the gift, may allow embalming and use of the body in funeral services. If the gift is of a part of a body, the donee, upon the death of the donor and before embalming, shall cause the part to be removed without unnecessary mutilation. After removal of the part, custody of the remainder of the body vests in the person under obligation to dispose of the body.

(b)   The time of death must be determined by a physician or surgeon who attends the donor at death or, if none, the physician or surgeon who certifies the death. Neither the physician or surgeon who attends the donor at death nor the physician or surgeon who determines the time of death may participate in the procedures for removing or transplanting a part unless the document of gift designates a particular physician or surgeon pursuant to Section 2(d).

(c)   If there has been an anatomical gift, a technician may remove any donated parts and an enucleator may remove any donated eyes or parts of eyes, after determination of death by a physician or surgeon.

SECTION 9.   COORDINATION OF PROCUREMENT AND USE.

Each hospital in this State, after consultation with other hospitals and procurement organizations, shall establish agreements or affiliations for coordination or procurement and use of human bodies and parts.

SECTION 10.   SALE OR PURCHASE OF PARTS PROHIBITED.

(a)   A person may not knowingly, for valuable consideration, purchase or sell a part for transplantation or therapy, if removal of the part is intended to occur after the death of the decedent.

(b)   Valuable consideration does not include reasonable payment for the removal, processing, disposal, preservation, quality control, storage, transportation, or implantation of a part.

(c)   A person who violates this section is guilty of a [felony] and upon conviction is subject to a fine not exceeding [$50,000] or imprisonment not exceeding [five] years, or both.

SECTION 11.   EXAMINATION, AUTOPSY, LIABILITY.

(a)   An anatomical gift authorizes any reasonable examination necessary to assure medical acceptability of the gift for the purposes intended.

(b)   The provisions of this [Act] are subject to the laws of this State governing autopsies.

(c)   A hospital, physician, surgeon, [coroner], [medical examiner], [local public health officer], enucleator, technician, or other person, who acts in accordance with this [Act] or with the applicable anatomical gift law of another state [or a foreign country] or attempts in good faith to do so is not liable for that act in a civil action or criminal proceeding.

(d)   An individual who makes an anatomical gift pursuant to Section 2 or 3 and the individual's estate are not liable for any injury or damage that may result from the making or the use of the anatomical gift.

SECTION 12. TRANSITIONAL PROVISIONS.

This [Act] applies to a document of gift, revocation, or refusal to make an anatomical gift signed by the donor or a person authorized to make or object to making an anatomical gift before, on, or after the effective date of this [Act].

SECTION 13. UNIFORMITY OF APPLICATION AND CONSTRUCTION.

This [Act] shall be applied and construed to effectuate its general purpose to make uniform the law with respect to the subject of this [Act] among states enacting it.

SECTION 14. SEVERABILITY.

If any provision of this [Act] or its application thereof to any person or circumstance is held invalid, the invalidity does not affect other provisions or applications of this [Act] which can be given effect without the invalid provision or application, and to this end the provisions of this [Act] are severable.

SECTION 15. SHORT TITLE.

This [Act] may be cited as the "Uniform Anatomical Gift Act (1987)."

SECTION 16. REPEALS.

The following acts and parts of acts are repealed:

(1)
(2)
(3)

SECTION 17. EFFECTIVE DATE.

This [Act] takes effect_____ .

SAMPLE ORGAN DONOR CARD

To receive an organ donor card, write Transplant International (Canada), P.O. Box 5339, London, Ontario N6A 5A5. Following are the front and back of the donor card.

TRANSPLANT
International (Canada)
Organ Donor's Next-of-Kin Identification
Identification du plus proche parent du donneur d'organes

I have discussed my wishes to be an organ donor with the person named below. In the event of my death, please contact:
J'ai parlé de mon désir d'être un donneur d'organes à la personne nommée ci-dessous. Advenant mon décès, veuillez contacter:

Name of next-of-kin
Nom du plus proche parent ...... Mrs ANGIE STILLER

Address
Adresse ......

City
Ville LONDON   Province
                                   Prov. ONTARIO

P.C.
C.P. ......   Telephone
                                   Téléphone ......

Back

ORGAN DONOR CARD
CARTE DE DONNEUR D'ORGANES

I/Je, soussigné(e) Calvin R STILLER
having attained the age of 18 years, consent to the use after my death of: (check appropriate choice)
étant âgé(e) de 18 ans ou plus, fais don après mon décès: (cochez la case appropriée)

A ☒ any needed organs or parts of my body
      de tout organe ou de toute partie de mon corps jugés utiles

B ☐ only the following organs or parts of my body:
      uniquement des organes suivants ou des parties suivantes de mon corps:

for transplant treatment, medical education or research.
pour transplantation, traitement, enseignement médical ou récherche médicale.

Signature of donor/*Signature du donneur*   Date/*Date* January 1/90

Front

INDEX

rights
    of donor, 92, 102, 108, 176
    of family, 92, 102, 108, 176

Sandoz Corporation, 24-25
Santamaria, Connie, 47
Saskatchewan Heart Fund, 52
Schneider, Andrew, 130, 132
Schouten, Fred and Karen, 144, 145
    baby Gabriel, 144, 145
shortness of breath, 50
Shumway, Norman, 4
siblings, living donations, 2, 19, 121-29
skin transplants, 20, 38
small bowel transplants, 20
Stanford University, California, 21
Starzl, Tom, 4, 21, 43
success rate, 80
    and cyclosporine, 21
    sibling donations, 19
    statistics, 19, 21, 27, 79, 170

Tadros, Nader, 48
technology, 19, 38, 73, 79, 172
    costs, 81
    and the future, 170-72
temperature
    for organ transportation, 33
    of recipient, 50
Terasaki, Paul, 43
T-helper cells, 22-24, 25-26, 27
TI. *See* Transplant International
time factor
    organ death, 29, 57, 89-91
    organ rejection, 23
    for types of transplants, 33
tissue typing, 2, 29, 122-24
training programs, 79, 81
Transplantation Society, 129-30, 133-35
transplant centers, 6, 8, 38, 67-70
    and staff morale, 68

and waiting list, 17-18, 62, 63-64, 67
transplant coordinators, 7, 8
    donor, 29, 33, 47
    recipient, 47, 50
Transplant International, 15, 52
transplant team, 29, 67, 68-70
    costs, 82
    and living donations, 130
    and recovery, 50
transplant units, 67-70, 95-96, 170
    costs, 81-82
    and hospital funding, 114-15
transplant waiting list, 52, 61-62, 114.
    See also organ sharing networks
    kidneys, 64-65
    registration, 63-64
transportation of organs, 29, 31, 33
    costs, 82
    temperature, 33
Truog, Robert, 143
24-ALERT, 7

Uniform Anatomical Gift Act, United
    States, 108
United Network for Organ Sharing
    (UNOS), 7, 65-66, 73
    urgency rating, 65
University Hospital, London, 3, 6, 12,
    21, 46-49, 56, 69, 77,
    111, 116, 118, 144, 161
UNOS. *See* United Network for Organ
    Sharing
urgency rating, 7-8, 65-66, 70, 72, 114

vegetative functions, 138-39, 140, 143
vegetative state, persistent, 142-43
Victoria Hospital, London, 2   *ONT. CANADA*

Wall, Bill, 118
weight gain, 50
White, David, 21, 26
wound healing, 69